When the Brain Can't Cope

When the Brain Can't Cope: Introducing Brain Fatigue Syndrome is a groundbreaking book pioneering the clinical condition of Brain Fatigue Syndrome, characterized by cognitive, emotional, and sensory impairment and profound exhaustion after mental activity that is not relieved by rest or sleep. It offers a thorough description, including its relationship to other pathologies and symptoms, method of study and recognition, and comprehensive management.

The book defines and describes brain fatigue, outlining how it can be assessed. Presenting a pathophysiological explanation at the cellular level, the authors also include research-based treatment strategies aimed at improving daily functioning and quality of life. To bring visibility to this often "invisible" condition, personal stories from individuals living with brain fatigue are incorporated, along with practical and real-life examples to raise awareness of the reality of this complex syndrome.

It is valuable reading for students of neuropsychology, medicine, nursing, and occupational therapy, as well as various healthcare professionals who work in the field of neurorehabilitation for acquired brain damage and those in primary care settings.

Birgitta Johansson is an associate professor and a clinical neuropsychologist at the University of Gothenburg and is also educated as a neurobiologist. In the clinic, her work with patients with brain injuries, strokes, and other neurological disorders has revealed brain fatigue to be a central problem. Consequently, our understanding of brain fatigue has developed, and the research we perform today enables clinical experience to be integrated with neurobiology and neuropsychology.

Lars Rönnbäck is a professor emeritus and a retired chief physician in neurology at the University of Gothenburg. He has focused extensively on glial cells, the support cells in the brain. His research has focused on developing a method to understand the signalling mechanisms between different types of brain cells, particularly between nerve cells and glial cells. As a result of this work, Lars Rönnbäck has formulated a hypothesis about the origin of brain fatigue, suggesting that glial deterioration, especially in the glutamate uptake capacity by astrocytes, plays a central role.

When the Brain Can't Cope
Introducing Brain Fatigue Syndrome

Birgitta Johansson and Lars Rönnbäck

Routledge
Taylor & Francis Group
LONDON AND NEW YORK

Cover image: Getty Images

First published 2026
by Routledge
4 Park Square, Milton Park, Abingdon, Oxon OX14 4RN

and by Routledge
605 Third Avenue, New York, NY 10158

Routledge is an imprint of the Taylor & Francis Group, an informa business

British Library Cataloguing-in-Publication Data
A catalogue record for this book is available from the British Library

ISBN: 978-1-041-22401-3 (hbk)
ISBN: 978-1-041-22400-6 (pbk)
ISBN: 978-1-003-73210-5 (ebk)

DOI: 10.4324/9781003732105

Typeset in Times New Roman
by SPi Technologies India Pvt Ltd (Straive)

Contents

Preface

Brain fatigue is a condition that many of us encounter, but few truly understand. This book delves into what we commonly call brain fatigue – a state of deep exhaustion resulting from illness or injury that depletes our energy reserves. Brain fatigue can occur for various reasons, including traumatic brain injuries, stroke, multiple sclerosis (MS), Parkinson's disease, brain tumours, meningitis, burnout syndrome, myalgic encephalomyelitis (ME), cancer due to the illness itself or treatment, and psychiatric disorders such as major depression, severe anxiety disorders, and schizophrenia. Even individuals with rheumatic diseases or endocrinological disorders, especially those with widespread inflammation in the body, including autoimmunity, often experience this debilitating fatigue.

People suffering from brain fatigue often experience accompanying symptoms such as emotional instability, sensitivity to sound and light, sensitivity to stress, difficulty initiating activities, and sleep problems.

We propose the term "Brain Fatigue Syndrome" as a collective name for this complex of symptoms. In this book, we aim to describe the individual symptoms, explain who can be affected, present a hypothesis underlying the symptoms at a cellular level, and propose an explanation for why the symptoms can become long-lasting. Furthermore, we explore diagnostic possibilities and provide examples of potential treatments.

The knowledge gap

Despite its prevalence, brain fatigue and its accompanying symptoms remain shrouded in obscurity. Our hope is that this book will bridge the knowledge gap and inspire further research on this topic. We draw on our extensive research, clinical experience, and the work of other experts in the field to provide a comprehensive understanding of brain fatigue. Through personal stories, we aim to offer deeper insights into this abstract phenomenon and foster curiosity and empathy.

The human experience

Many individuals living with Brain Fatigue Syndrome face frustration and shame due to a lack of understanding from themselves, their families, friends, and even healthcare providers. They often set unrealistic expectations for themselves, which can be detrimental to their well-being. This book seeks to shed light on their experiences and provide practical strategies for managing brain fatigue.

Healthcare

Many patients seek healthcare support for brain fatigue. Today, Brain fatigue can be alleviated, and we present examples of treatment alternatives that may be useful. Support may be needed periodically, as the recovery process is often prolonged.

Target audience

This book is designed for a wide audience, including healthcare students (future doctors, nurses, psychologists, occupational therapists, physiotherapists, and speech therapists), current healthcare professionals, and those involved in municipal activities such as home care and housing support. We also address authorities such as the Social Insurance Agency and Insurance Companies. Of course, we also turn to those affected, their relatives, and anyone else who wants in-depth knowledge and understanding.

Introducing the authors

The authors, Birgitta Johansson, associate professor and clinical neuropsychologist, and Lars Rönnbäck, senior professor and former chief physician in neurology, both at Sahlgrenska Academy, University of Gothenburg, and Sahlgrenska University Hospital in Gothenburg, Sweden, have long worked with research and in the hospital with people who suffer from brain fatigue.

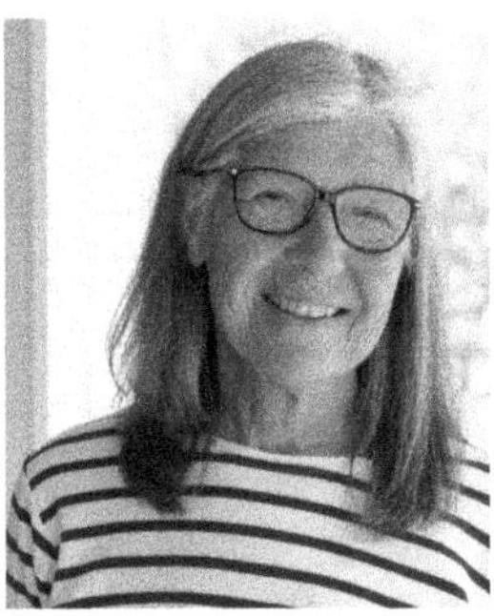

Birgitta Johansson has worked for a long time with rehabilitation after acquired brain injuries and, in parallel, with research on brain fatigue following acquired brain injuries. Her driving force is to provide those affected with help and support. Spreading knowledge about brain fatigue is of high priority.

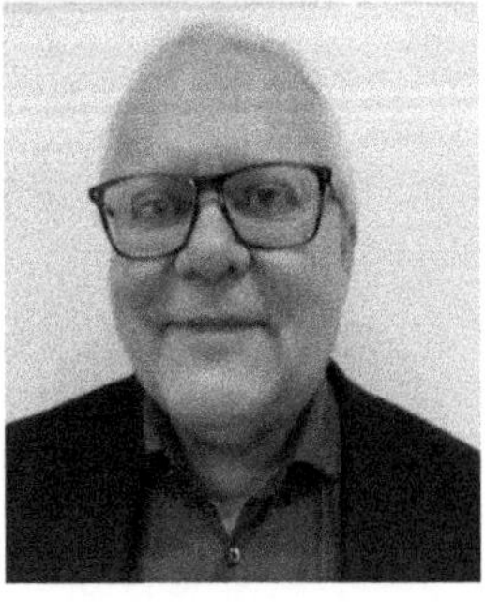

Lars Rönnbäck is interested in the signalling between the brain's astrocytes and how these cells affect communication between nerve cells. It is, among other things, studies of this type that form the basis for a hypothesis of the Brain Fatigue Syndrome presented in the book.

The clinical work we have both undertaken, along with our research, has contributed to the systematization and structuring of our understanding of brain fatigue. The countless encounters with patients in the clinic and with participants in studies, their stories, and the study results have collectively given us deeper insight into the problems that brain fatigue entails. We have both been deeply involved in all the studies we describe in the book, from design to report writing. It has become clear to us how different treatments can be helpful, though not curative. We have written many articles ranging from cell biology to the treatment of brain fatigue, but much knowledge is still missing, and research on brain fatigue, its origins, and treatment needs to be intensified. With this book, we aim to convey the deep and broad knowledge we have about brain fatigue and why we are introducing the concept of Brain Fatigue Syndrome. We hope this book will contribute to increased understanding and knowledge about brain fatigue.

Illustrations

Verity Tolcher created the illustrations for the book. She has a degree in Product Design from Edinburgh Napier University and a Master of Design from Auckland University of Technology.

The other figures in the book were produced by Birgitta Johansson, all based on the research she has participated in.

1 What is fatigue?

Fatigue is a state affecting all people in daily life, and we all need to rest and sleep regularly, which is the foundation for good health. However, in our hectic society, many suffer from fatigue, and it is one of the most common reasons for people to seek primary care.

Studies have revealed a significant discrepancy in opinions regarding the importance of acknowledging fatigue between medical doctors and patients. In a study conducted many years ago, it was found that among individuals seeking medical care for fatigue and perceiving it as a significant issue, doctors did not always take the fatigue as seriously as the patients did. Many patients experience the same thing even today. One explanation could be that fatigue does not have to be a sign of illness. Fatigue can have several causes, such as sleep problems, stress, mild depression, and pain. Different medications can also cause fatigue, and sometimes, different factors, including social problems, work together. It may therefore be understandable that fatigue may be considered a minor problem if the doctor does not find signs of illness requiring treatment. This may also be explained by the lack of consensus in defining and assessing fatigue.

Fatigue is a private experience and is often not externally visible. It can neither be detected nor quantified by a blood sample or other test. After a heavy workday, a hard test at school, or not sleeping well, most people experience fatigue. This fatigue is of a temporary nature, and after some rest and good sleep, life is back to normal.

The endurance is restricted

The fatigue discussed in this book affects people's whole lives, reducing their ability to work and participate in social activities, and is not restored after some days of rest and healthy sleep. It may improve slightly after a longer rest, but the person will still be easily exhausted while doing mental

DOI: 10.4324/9781003732105-1

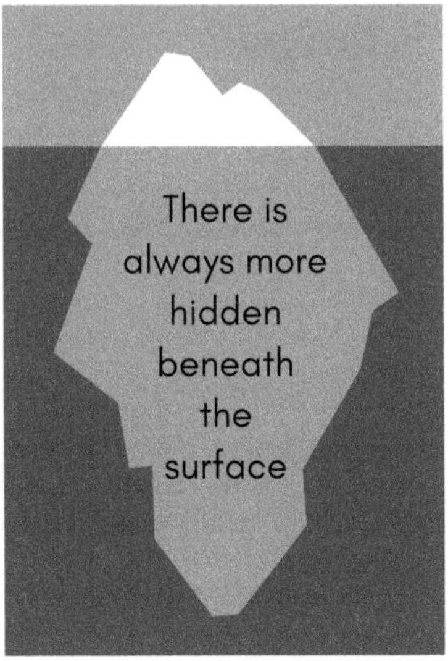

Figure 1.1 The invisible fatigue.

activities, such as taking part in a conversation, and experiencing shortcomings in mental functioning, such as concentration and memory difficulties. This specific fatigue is about the inherent inability to be mentally active over time, limiting how long and how often activities can be performed. The endurance is restricted. It is about how consistently and for how long ordinary activities can be done without experiencing profound exhaustion. This fatigue is far beyond and far deeper than what a healthy person can understand. It can be compared to an iceberg, with the main part being invisible below the surface. Even if we can't see or clearly understand the impact the unseen can have on life, we must learn and take it into account; otherwise, we can get into trouble (Figure 1.1).

Fatigue can be compared to an iceberg. What is visible above the surface is only a small part of the whole. The unseen depths must be understood to grasp the full impact.

The experience of this specific fatigue is common in several diseases, especially those affecting the nervous system. For example, many medical professionals and non-professionals believe that disturbances in motor, sensory, or coordination functions are the most disabling symptoms of multiple sclerosis (MS), but it is often the fatigue that is considered by the patient to be the worst symptom. The same is true after a stroke or a traumatic brain injury (TBI), especially for those who are well recovered.

For a long time, we have worked with research and in the hospital with patients who suffer from reduced mental energy. We have developed diagnostic instruments, performed treatment studies, and are particularly interested in the origin of this specific fatigue and how people can get relief and be understood. We are launching the new name Brain Fatigue Syndrome, or short brain fatigue, and will in this book present a theoretical model, the symptom complex, and possible treatment options for alleviating brain fatigue.

The Brain Fatigue Syndrome

In research and clinical practice, we encounter terms like fatigue, physical fatigue, stroke-fatigue, MS-fatigue, brain fog, cognitive fatigue, central fatigue, neurological fatigue, post-concussion syndrome, and chronic fatigue. Additionally, there is no consensus in defining fatigue and no golden standard to assess it, all with a risk that fatigue is not acknowledged. It is complicated and invisible.

Chaudhuri and Behan defined central fatigue as difficulty in initiating and sustaining voluntary activities, not as muscle weakness or depression (Chaudhuri & Behan, 2004). They summed up with the statement that

> To imply that fatigue is a medically unexplained, non-organic symptom in patients who do not have a primary psychiatric diagnosis would be incorrect and inappropriate. As in other complex medical disorders, only open-minded people who are willing to consider observations and explanations at many different levels are likely to succeed in offering the right solutions.

We agree with this statement. We need to be open-minded, listen to patients, and be curious in the struggle to improve knowledge and treatment options.

We initially chose the term "mental fatigue" to distinguish it from physical fatigue. Later, we added "pathological" to mental fatigue to differentiate the pathological mental fatigue we discuss from the normal mental fatigue everyone can experience after intense mental activity.

Fatigue is also suggested to be divided into state and trait fatigue. State fatigue refers to reduced performance in a test over a specified time, called fatigability, or an increased perception of fatigue in relation to a specific activity performed, often measured with a visual analogue scale. Trait fatigue is measured with assessment scales as the subjective perception of fatigue the person experiences over a predefined period, such as weeks or months.

To address the confusion surrounding fatigue terminology, we introduce the term Brain Fatigue Syndrome. This conclusion stems from extensive research and clinical experience with various diseases affecting the brain. We want to emphasize the origin of fatigue from the brain and the symptom cluster involved, including cognitive, emotional, and sensory aspects, all closely related to the extreme exhaustion that cannot be alleviated by rest and sleep. From now on, we will refer to this condition as Brain Fatigue Syndrome, or simply brain fatigue.

> **Brain Fatigue Syndrome** emphasizes the origin of fatigue from the brain and the symptom cluster involved, including cognitive, emotional, and sensory aspects, all closely related to the extreme exhaustion that cannot be alleviated by rest and sleep.

For assessing the Brain Fatigue Syndrome, we have used the Mental Fatigue Scale (MFS) for various diagnostic groups over a long period. It has become clear to us that Brain Fatigue Syndrome occurs across multiple diagnostic groups, here illustrated in Figure 1.2 with acquired brain injury (mild TBI, TBI, stroke), hypothyroidism, Graves' disease (hyperthyroidism), and burnout syndrome (BOS). Affected individuals report

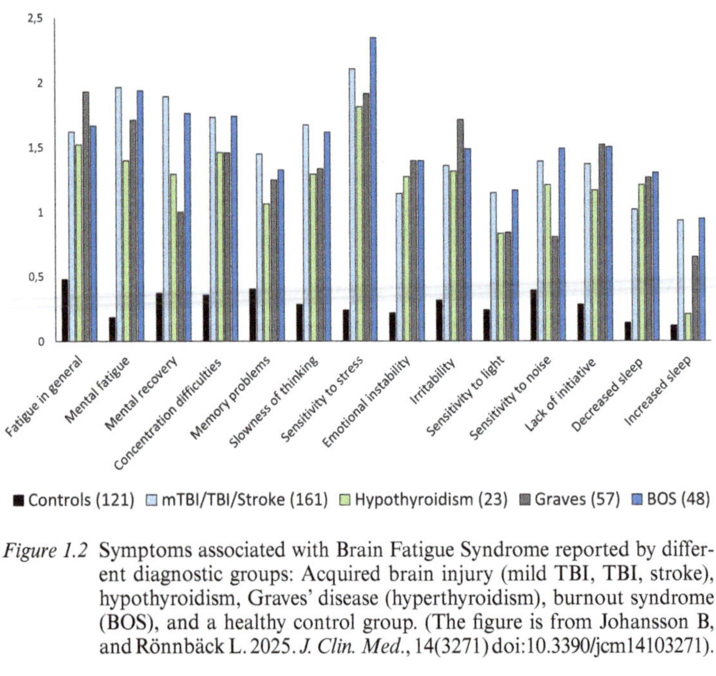

Figure 1.2 Symptoms associated with Brain Fatigue Syndrome reported by different diagnostic groups: Acquired brain injury (mild TBI, TBI, stroke), hypothyroidism, Graves' disease (hyperthyroidism), burnout syndrome (BOS), and a healthy control group. (The figure is from Johansson B, and Rönnbäck L. 2025. *J. Clin. Med.*, 14(3271) doi:10.3390/jcm14103271).

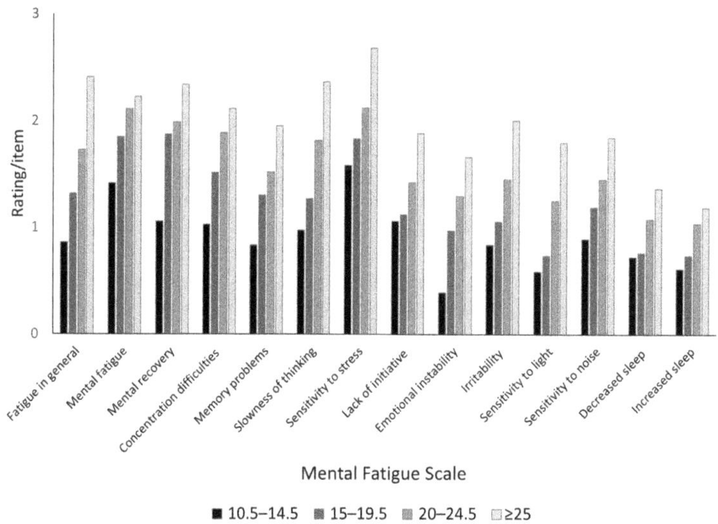

Figure 1.3 Symptoms associated with Brain Fatigue Syndrome, as measured by the Mental Fatigue Scale (MFS), among participants with acquired brain injury (including traumatic brain injury and stroke). Total MFS scores are divided into four severity levels (10.5–14.5, 15–19.5, 20–24.5, and ≥25). The figure shows how symptom ratings vary across these levels, with higher scores indicating more severe symptoms across all categories.

remarkably similar symptoms when their scores exceed the cutoff. For comparison, a healthy control group is shown.

Figure 1.3 demonstrates how all symptoms associated with Brain Fatigue Syndrome are closely interconnected and tend to vary in concert with the level of fatigue experienced. This is shown by dividing MFS scores into four severity levels (10.5–14.5, 15–19.5, 20–20.5, and ≥25). For example, when concentration decreases, noise sensitivity and irritability typically increase, among other symptoms described in detail later in this book. Despite differences in terminology across conditions, the MFS reliably detects Brain Fatigue Syndrome.

A personal journey. From a head injury (concussion) to long-lasting Brain Fatigue Syndrome

In mid-November 2017, I went out to the paddock to refill the hay for the horses. My four-year-old mare, who is very curious and social, was the first to approach as usual. This time, she came a bit too close, so I asked her to back up to make room for the hay net. That's the last thing

I remember. When I woke up, I was lying on the ground, and the throbbing pain in my head made it clear what had happened. "No, not a concussion again," I thought to myself. I had already had a concussion earlier that year and had been bedridden for over a week. "I don't have time for this," was my next thought. Summer 2017 was the year I realized my big dream, owning my own horse farm, so I had a lot to do.

I got help to stand up but immediately had to sit down on the edge of the paddock; I was too dizzy and slightly nauseous. Later, when I looked in the mirror, I saw a clear hoof print in the mud on my cap where the kick had hit, right at my temple.

The doctors confirmed that I had a concussion, a physical trauma. I was told to go home and rest. Since I had had concussions several times before, both as an adult and as a child, the condition was not entirely unfamiliar to me. Despite this, the frustration of not being able to be productive kept growing worse. My sick leave was extended repeatedly, and I began to wonder why I never got better. The progress in my recovery was so small compared to the significant setbacks I faced whenever I overexerted myself. It felt like something was wrong. It usually doesn't take this long to recover!

As I write this, about a year and two months since the accident, I am still not well. Several doctor visits and various tests and investigations have led to a diagnosis of post-concussion syndrome. They call it fatigue in medical terms, or brain fatigue in Swedish. The hardest part right now is accepting the situation as it is. I work on this every day, dealing with my frustration over not functioning normally. Fatigue and headaches are a handicap I may have to live with for the rest of my life, and that is hard to accept. I have always been a person with many irons in the fire, whether it's about hobbies, interests, or work. The otherwise social person I consider myself to be now constantly must limit the events I attend to avoid overexertion. Everyday activities like having coffee with friends, spending time with my nieces and nephews, and other family members are incredibly exhausting, and I constantly have to remind myself not to plan too many activities in one day. Too much stimulation and intense sensory impressions cause setbacks, sometimes immediately and sometimes a few days later. Life has become harder to plan. I always feel uneasy about having to keep plans open and not being able to give definitive answers to invitations because I might need to cancel if I'm not feeling well. In most cases, I can't fully participate in parties, family dinners, or follow interesting discussions or TV programs. I fear being misunderstood, that people might think I refuse or leave early because I don't want to participate, or that they might stop inviting me because I often can't manage. But the times I do manage to be there are so valuable and important to me. It's a sorrow not to be able to participate; my will is not the issue. In between, frustration comes in various forms, often in tears and sadness when I'm alone.

Returning to my profession as a high school teacher has been tough. After initially being on full-time sick leave, I gradually managed to work half-time. This is a significant achievement for me, but it hasn't been easy. Through a rehab course, I, along with others in similar situations, have learned to conserve energy. It's very difficult but necessary to complete the workday. Without the lessons from the course, I probably wouldn't have managed to increase my work hours. The fact that the Swedish Social Insurance Agency does not accept the doctors' certificates and medical assessments makes recovery harder, rather the opposite. Since it has been over a year, they now want me to work full-time (regardless of the job) even though the doctors say it goes against the rehabilitation plan and is a health risk. Being cut off from insurance is incredibly stressful on many levels. I want nothing more than to function normally and return to full-time work. But during this time, I have realized that my life is more important than any job in the world. I don't want and can't risk crashing by forcing myself to work one hundred percent. Not when I have come this far. There must be other ways.

The maxillofacial surgeon I was referred to because my left jaw was misaligned from the kick has repeatedly told me that I should be glad I survived; he says it is more common not to survive such a blow. And I am, of course. Deep down, I'm glad my horse wasn't shod on the hind hooves that day in November, though on my worst days, I sometimes think it would have been better if she had kicked me to death.

The elusive brain fatigue

Brain fatigue is an abstract phenomenon that is difficult to understand both for the sufferer and for those around them. When meeting people who suffer from brain fatigue, at first glance, they seem like anyone else. So how can it be possible to understand what cannot be seen and felt? How can the extreme fatigue that the person experiences, perhaps only after a short conversation, and the lack of energy in most everyday situations, as well as the long recovery needed, be understood? Brain fatigue is thus not an ordinary fatigue or sleepiness that everyone can perceive in the evening. It is not the fatigue we can feel in the body when we have performed a physical activity, nor is it the temporary mental tiredness that can occur after a longer mental activity. Brain fatigue is instead an extreme lack of mental energy that does not disappear after rest.

The affected person can often do everything in the present moment; the function exists, but when the energy runs out, the person cannot continue. After that, it can be difficult to think clearly; it doesn't work to pay attention to more than one thing at a time, more mistakes can be made, and rest is needed. However, most people slow down their speed in favour of doing things right, if possible. But sometimes, the pace is not possible to adjust, as in following a conversation or the hectic traffic.

Another important factor is the sensitivity to impressions, such as seeing and hearing. This is commonly regarded as highly difficult to manage, and they can describe this as being overwhelmed with impressions and unable to filter redundant information away. The person may choose not to join colleagues in the coffee room and instead prefer a quiet environment, risking being considered as not willing to connect with other people. The music in the restaurant can be totally unbearable, or the fan in the background. We will come back to this later. However, today's fast-paced society gives rise to a lot of impressions, unconscious and conscious, and everything is registered by the brain. The personal story illustrates this.

We can conclude that most people who suffer from brain fatigue are gifted and have great ambition, and they are not lazy.

Personal story. It is difficult to understand

> I'm starting to realize that I push myself too much. This became very clear to me the other day at work. About 50 of us gathered in the dining hall for speeches and songs. It was delightful! But I quickly felt overwhelmed, even though I wanted to be there. I had seated myself on the edge to avoid being in the middle of the crowd.
>
> Then, a colleague approached me and gently asked if she could take my seat because she wears two hearing aids and all the noise is amplified, making it hard for her to hear. Of course, I agreed and made space for her. At that moment, it hit me, this is exactly how it feels for me too, like all the sounds are being sucked in and I can't hear anything, just a cacophony of noise everywhere!
>
> I stayed at the event for about an hour, but when I left, I literally walked away with a headache. It lingered and became this relentless torment that's hard to describe, no painkiller can alleviate it. I just had to endure it, all Friday, all Saturday, and half of Sunday. Not being able to watch TV or read newspapers. I can live with, but not being able to interact and be social, that truly makes me suffer.

Who may suffer from Brain Fatigue Syndrome?

Brain fatigue can be a consequence of damage or disease in the nervous system. For most people, the fatigue disappears as the injury or illness heals. For others, the brain fatigue remains for months or years or even becomes chronic. Brain fatigue can occur after a traumatic head injury (TBI), mild to severe, including concussion, a stroke, even a mild transient stroke such as TIA (transient ischaemic attack), meningitis, encephalitis, cardiac arrest with effects on the brain, brain tumour, cerebral palsy (CP), multiple sclerosis (MS), Parkinson's disease, and many other neurological diseases. Endocrine diseases can also cause long-term problems with brain fatigue. Brain fatigue is also present after severe and prolonged stress, such as burnout syndrome, in myalgic encephalomyelitis (ME)/chronic fatigue syndrome, and post-COVID and from cancer itself or its treatment. People suffering from neuropsychiatric disabilities such as Attention-Deficit/Hyperactivity Disorder

(ADHD) and autism, psychiatric diseases such as major depression, anxiety, and schizophrenia, as well as people with inflammatory system

Table 1.1 Examples of common diseases and conditions that often give rise to brain fatigue for children and adults

• Stroke	• Cardiac arrest
• Traumatic brain injury	• Endocrine disorders
• Meningitis and encephalitis	• Burnout syndrome
• Multiple sclerosis (MS)	• ME/Chronic fatigue
• Parkinson's disease	• Neuropsychiatric disorders as ADHD, autism
• Cerebral palsy (CP)	• Rheumatic disorders
• Brain tumour	• General inflammatory disorders
• Other neurological and psychiatric disorders	

diseases such as rheumatic disease (RA) or systemic lupus erythematosus (SLE), often suffer from brain fatigue. Although other symptoms often dominate in ongoing diseases of the nervous system or systemic diseases, brain fatigue may not get the attention it deserves (Table 1.1).

All ages can suffer

Brain fatigue affects people of all ages. Adults can often describe the difference between their condition before and after the illness or injury more clearly. Children and adolescents also suffer from brain fatigue, but it can be more challenging for them to articulate the problem, especially if they have lived with the illness from birth. Their rapidly changing lives due to development can also make it harder to describe. For example, it is becoming increasingly clear that brain fatigue exists in individuals with cerebral palsy. While adults report it, knowledge about its impact on children and teenagers is limited. Even the elderly report pathological brain fatigue after diseases.

Diagnostic groups

We are fully aware that brain fatigue can occur in various diseases or after brain damage. However, we will often refer to traumatic brain injuries, strokes, and neurological diseases, as these are the diagnostic groups where we have conducted most of our research. As a neurologist in a neurological clinic and a neuropsychologist in a rehabilitation medicine clinic, we have also encountered several other diagnostic groups with neurological diseases. Over the years, we have met and listened to many patients who have shared their stories, problems, and life situations when suffering from brain fatigue.

In addition, we have collaborated with researchers working with endocrinological patients, where brain fatigue is also present. Our experience indicates that Brain Fatigue Syndrome exists across various diagnostic groups, as evidenced by ratings above the cutoff on the Mental Fatigue Scale (MFS). These ratings reveal very similar symptoms regardless of the disease, even if the causes differ, as shown in Figure 1.2 with brain injury, stress, or endocrine disorder.

How many suffer from Brain Fatigue Syndrome?

We do not know for sure how many people suffer from long-term brain fatigue after neurological diseases. After a mild head injury, such as a concussion, the majority recover within a few weeks or months, but not all. Research reports indicate that 10–70% of those who have had a head injury suffer from fatigue for a few years, up to 10 years, or even lifelong. After a stroke, about 36–77% suffer from fatigue, in Parkinson's disease, 28–58%, and in multiple sclerosis, 38–83%. These varying figures reflect the difficulty and discrepancy in assessing fatigue, as different assessment scales are used. However, the figures are higher than in the general population, where fatigue is estimated to be present in 5–20% of people.

Some have problems to a lesser degree and cope with everyday work and social activities quite well, but not perfectly, and struggle with reduced activity levels, especially with work. Others have severe problems and are unable to work.

Brain Fatigue Syndrome in relation to activity

Brain fatigue is affected by daily activities and the type of activities performed. A person who works full-time may report just as severe problems with brain fatigue as someone who is on full-time sick leave. Therefore, the rating scale and the symptoms described must always be understood in relation to the person's activity level and overall life situation.

Brain Fatigue Syndrome in relation to injury severity

When comparing individuals who have had a milder or more severe head injury or stroke, the person with the more severe injury may, after a few years, have very similar problems with brain fatigue as someone who has suffered a milder brain injury. Why is this the case? We do not have a definitive answer, but we will discuss this in the theoretical part of this book.

Why does Brain Fatigue Syndrome last?

Experiencing brain fatigue immediately after a head injury, stroke, or other brain disease is understandable for most people. But why does brain fatigue become long-lasting in some individuals even after the injury or disease appears to have healed? Currently, there is no clear explanation for this. In chronic disorders like multiple sclerosis and Parkinson's disease, it is easier to understand, but why does brain fatigue persist after a mild stroke or concussion/mild TBI? A hypothetical explanation could be that astrocytes remain in an inflammatory-reactive state. More about this will be discussed later in this book.

Bibliography

Asher, A., Fu, J. B., Bailey, C., & Hughes, J. K. (2016). Fatigue among patients with brain tumors. *CNS Oncology*, 5(2), 91–100.

Askari, S., Harvey, K., & Sam-Odutola, M. (2024). Patients experience of cognitive fatigue post-stroke: An exploratory study. *Disability and Rehabilitation*, 46(19), 4514–4521. https://doi.org/10.1080/09638288.2023.2280065

Barbek, R., Makowski, A. C., & von dem Knesebeck, O. (2025). Perceived discrimination in fatigue: A qualitative interview study in the SOMA.SOC project. *Frontiers in Sociology*, 10. https://doi.org/10.3389/fsoc.2025.1528312

Beaulieu-Bonneau, S., & Ouellet, M.-C. (2017). Fatigue in the first year after traumatic brain injury: Course, relationship with injury severity, and correlates. *Neuropsychology Rehabilitation*, 27(7), 983–1001. https://doi.org/10.1080/09602011.2016.1162176

Bergqvist, L., Öhrvall, A.-M., Rönnbäck, L., Johansson, B., Himmelmann, K., & Peny-Dahlstrand, M. (2019). Evidence of construct validity for the modified mental fatigue scale when used in persons with cerebral palsy. *Developmental Neurorehabilitation*, 23(4), 240–252. https://doi.org/10.1080/17518423.2019.1645227

Bushnik, T., Englander, J., & Wright, J. (2008). The experience of fatigue in the first 2 years after moderate-to-severe traumatic brain injury: A preliminary report. *Journal of Head Trauma Rehabilitation*, 23(1), 17–24.

Cantor, J. B., Ashman, T., Gordon, W., Ginsberg, A., Engmann, C., Egan, M., . . . Flanagan, S. (2008). Fatigue after traumatic brain injury and its impact on participation and quality of life. *Journal of Head Trauma Rehabilitation*, 23(1), 41–51.

Cantor, J. B., Gordon, W., & Gumber, S. (2013). What is post TBI fatigue? *Neuropsychology Rehabilitation*, 32, 875–883.

Chaudhuri, A., & Behan, P. O. (2004). Fatigue in neurological disorders. *Lancet*, 363, 978–988.

Danson, E., Brunsdon, R., Lane-Brown, A., & Oxenham, V. (2025). A cognitive energy crisis: A systematic review & meta-analysis of effective interventions for pediatric cognitive fatigue post-acquired brain injury. *Neuropsychological Rehabilitation*, 11, 1–26. https://doi.org/10.1080/09602011.2025.2540625

Diaz-Arias, L. A., Yeshokumar, A. K., Glassberg, B., Sumowski, J. F., Easton, A., Probasco, J. C., & Venkatesan, A. (2021). Fatigue in survivors of autoimmune encephalitis. *Neurology Neuroimmunology & Neuroinflammation*, 8, 6. https://doi.org/10.1212/NXI.0000000000001064

Dohrenwend, B., & Crandell, D. (1970). Psychiatric symptoms in community, clinic and mental hospital groups. *American Journal of Psychiatry*, 126, 1611–1621.

Eng, J. J., Bird, M.-L., Godecke, E., Hoffmann, T. C., Laurin, C., Olaoye, O. A., . . . Walker, M. F. (2019). Moving stroke rehabilitation research evidence into clinical practice: Consensus-based core recommendations from the stroke recovery and rehabilitation roundtable. *Neurorehabilitation and Neural Repair*, 33(11), 935–942. https://doi.org/10.1177/1545968319886485

Eriksson, G., Larsson, I., Guidetti, S., & Johansson, U. (2023). Handling fatigue in everyday activities at five years after stroke: A long and demanding process. *Scandinavian Journal of Occupational Therapy*, February;30(2), 228–238. https://doi.org/10.1080/11038128.2022.2089230

Fahrenfort, J. J., Wilterdink, A. M. L., & van der Veen, E. A. (2000). Long-term residual complaints and psychosocial sequelae after remission of hyperthyroidism. *Psychoneuroendocrinology*, 25, 201–211.

Finley, C. R., Chan, D. S., Garrison, S., Korownyk, C., Kolber, M. R., Campbell, S., . . . Allan, M. (2018). What are the most common conditions in primary care? Systematic review. *Canadian Family Physician*, 64, 832–840.

Friedman, J. H., Brown, R. G., Comella, C., Garber, C. E., Krupp, L. B., Lou, J.-S., . . . Taylor, B. (2007). Fatigue in Parkinsons's disease: A review. *Movement Disorders*, 22(3), 297–308.

Hinkle, J. L., Becker, K. J., Kim, J. S., Choi-Kwon, S., Saban, K. L., McNair, N., & Mead, G. E. (2017). Poststroke fatigue: Emerging evidence and approaches to management: A scientific statement for healthcare professionals from the American Heart Association. *Stroke*, 48, e159–170.

Irestorm, E., Tonning Olsson, I., Johansson, B., & Øra, I. (2020). Cognitive fatigue in relation to depressive symptoms after treatment for childhood cancer. *BMC Psychology*, 8(1), 31.

Johansson, B., Berglund, P., & Rönnbäck, L. (2009). Mental fatigue and impaired information processing after mild and moderate traumatic brain injury. *Brain Injury*, 23(13–14), 1027–1040.

Johansson, B., Holmberg, M., Skau, S., Malmgren, H., & Filipsson Nyström, H. (2023). The relationship between mental fatigue, depression, and cognition in Graves' disease. *European Thyroid Journal*, 12(4), e230040. https://doi.org/10.1530/ETJ-23-0040

Johansson, B., & Rönnbäck, L. (2014). Evaluation of the mental fatigue scale and its relation to cognitive and emotional functioning after traumatic brain injury or stroke. *International Journal of Physical Medicine and Rehabilitation*, 2, 182. https://doi.org/10.4172/2329-9096.1000182

Johansson, B., & Rönnbäck, L. (2025). The brain fatigue syndrome—Symptoms, probable definition, and pathophysiological mechanisms. *Journal of Clinical Medicine*, 14(3271). https://doi.org/10.3390/jcm14103271

Joshi, V. L., Tang, L. H., Mikkelsen, T. B., Nielsen, J. F., Zinckernagel, L., Borregaard, B., . . . Zwisler, A.-D. (2023). Does time heal fatigue, psychological, cognitive and disability problems in people who experience an out-of-hospital cardiac arrest? Results from the DANCAS survey study. *Resuscitation*, 182, 109639.

Juengst, S., Skidmore, E., Arenth, P. M., Niyonkuru, C., & Raina, K. D. (2013). The unique contribution of fatigue to disability in community dwelling adults with traumatic brain injury. *Archives of Physical Medicine and Rehabilitation*, 94(1), 74–79.

Kluger, B. M., Krupp, L. B., & Enoka, R. M. (2013). Fatigue and fatigability in neurologic illnesses. Proposal for a unified taxonomy. *Neurology*, 80(4), 409–416.

Korte, S. M., & Straub, R. H. (2019). Fatigue in inflammatory rheumatic disorders: Pathophysiological mechanisms *Rheumatology*, 58(Suppl 5), 35–50. https://doi.org/10.1093/rheumatology/kez413

Krupp, L. B., Alvarez, L. A., LaRocca, N. G., & Scheinberg, L. C. (1988). Fatigue in multiple sclerosis. *Archives of Neurology*, 45, 435–437.

Palm, S., Rönnbäck, L., & Johansson, B. (2017). Long-term mental fatigue after traumatic brain injury and impact on capacity for work employment status. *Journal of Rehabilitation Medicine*, 49, (228–233).

Raymaker, D. A., Teo, A. R., Steckler, N. A., Lentz, B., Scharer, M., Santos, A. D., . . . Nicolaidis, C. (2020). "Having all of your internal resources exhausted beyond measure and being left with no clean-up crew": Defining autistic burnout. *Autism in Adulthood*, 2(2). https://doi.org/10.1089/aut.2019.0079

Samuelsson, C., Gunnarsson, L.-G., Svärdman, F., Rück, C., & Lindsäte, E. (2025). Physicians' experiences of assessing and supporting fatigued patients in primary care: A focus group study. *BMC Primary Care*, 26(197). https://doi.org/10.1186/s12875-025-02891-1

Staub, F., & Bogousslavsky, J. (2001). Fatigue after stroke: A major but neglected issue. *Cerebrovascular Diseases*, 12(2), 75–81.

Western, E., Nordenmark, T. H., Sorteberg, W., Karic, T., & Sorteberg, A. (2021). Fatigue after aneurysmal subarachnoid hemorrhage: Clinical characteristics and associated factors in patients with good outcome. *Frontiers in Behavioral Neuroscience*, 15, 633616. https://doi.org/10.3389/fnbeh.2021.633616

Zielinski, M. R., Systrom, D. M., & Rose, N. R. (2019). Fatigue, sleep, and autoimmune and related disorders. *Frontiers in Immunology*, 10, 1827. https://doi.org/10.3389/fimmu.2019.01827

2 Definition and common symptoms of Brain Fatigue Syndrome

Specific to the Brain Fatigue Syndrome is the reduced endurance for cognitive and social activities, work, studies, and for some, even after physical activities. All this results in reduced work ability and quality of life. Brain Fatigue Syndrome emanates from the brain, showing up with symptoms including cognitive, emotional, and sensory difficulties. All symptoms are closely related to the extreme exhaustion not possible to get rid of after rest and sleep. According to the theory of Brain Fatigue Syndrome, no specific anatomical area is central, and no specific area has so far been recognized to be related to it. We suggest that the Brain Fatigue Syndrome is due to a general effect on the brain with a dysfunction in brain cells (neurones and glia). That is why we define brain fatigue as a syndrome with closely connected symptoms, all emanating from dysfunction in brain cells and resulting for the afflicted in extreme fatigue.

Definition of Brain Fatigue Syndrome

We define Brain Fatigue Syndrome as an extreme lack of energy that manifests itself after mental activities, the more extensive the worse, it must have lasted at least one month, not being cured with rest and sleep, with a sum of scores above 10 on the Mental Fatigue Scale (read about MFS in the chapter of assessment), and include typical and associated symptoms (Figure 2.1).

Typical symptoms

- An unusual drain of mental energy upon mental activity.
- Impaired attention and concentration over time.
- Following over-exertion, a long recovery time disproportionate to the exertion level.
- Diurnal variation of the fatigue symptom, with the fatigue often being better in the mornings and worse in the afternoons and evenings. Often variations from one day to the next.

DOI: 10.4324/9781003732105-2

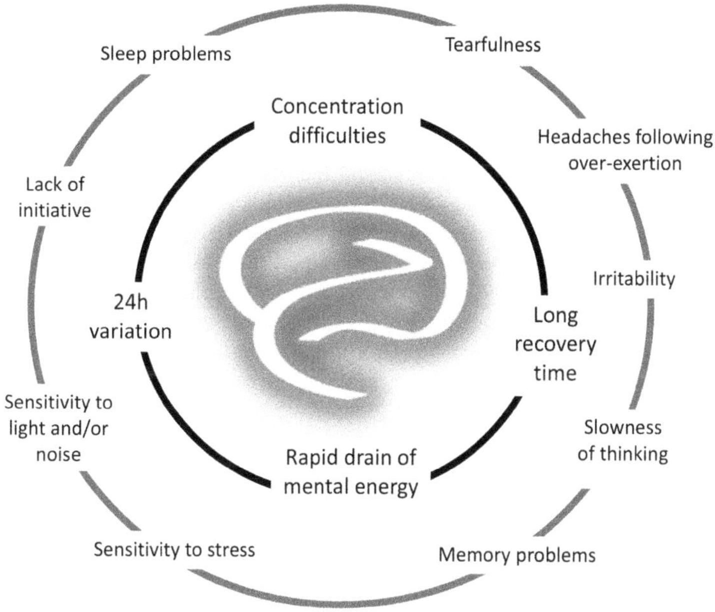

Figure 2.1 The Brain Fatigue Syndrome includes the central (inner circle) and associated symptoms (outer circle) with cognitive, emotional, sensory sensitivity, and sleep problems.

Associated symptoms

- Memory problems
- Slowness of thinking
- Reduced initiative
- Increased tendency to become emotional/tearfulness
- Irritability
- Stress sensitivity
- Sleep problems
- Sensitivity to, or intolerance of, light and noise
- Headaches following overexertion

When brain fatigue is most pronounced

Situations where brain fatigue often manifests itself are when being mentally active, as at work and in studies, but also during less demanding activities as reading a book or newspaper, being in conversations with people, during unforeseen events and situations with a lot of impressions, as in messy and noisy environments, e.g., shopping centres and public transport.

What living with brain fatigue can be like

For an outsider, it is most often very difficult to understand how a person with brain fatigue functions and how it is perceived. In short, brain fatigue can be compared with an old rechargeable battery or an old mobile phone with a bad battery. The person discharges quickly and needs a long time for recharge (Figure 2.2). The person has less energy already from the beginning in the morning and needs to economize the limited amount of energy available for the day, and there is no energy reserve.

Another comparison is a car with a small fuel tank and an inefficient engine. If you are "easy on the accelerator", drive the car carefully and stop at every gas station and refuel the car, you will be fine. If, on the other hand, you press hard on the accelerator and do not stop refuelling the car, you will suddenly run out of fuel, and the car will stop. Or we can relate to the electric car with the need to charge regularly. In the same way, a person suffering from brain fatigue needs to plan the activity and recharge or take pauses and rest regularly, and if not do that, they will become totally exhausted, and they can lose the ability to think and act.

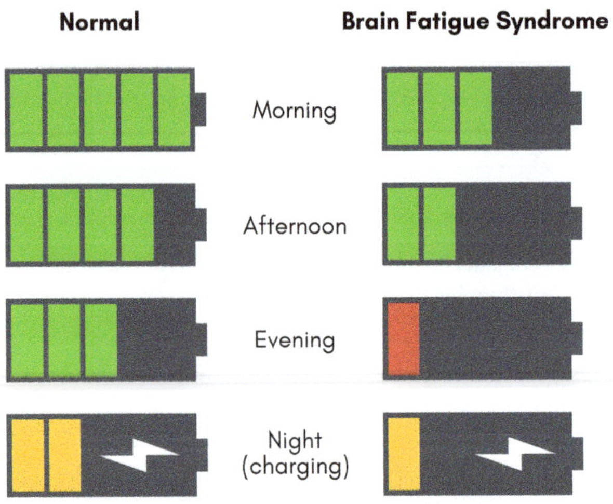

Figure 2.2 Illustration of, to the left, a non-brain-fatigued person. The battery is charged in the morning, and the energy is used during the day. At the end of the day, some extra energy exists. Recharging takes place during sleep. The batteries to the right illustrate the energy a brain-fatigued person has. There is a reduced amount of energy already in the morning, not fully charged, and the battery consumes the energy rapidly during the day. Depending on activities performed, the energy can be used up very quickly, or an extra charge during daytime may be necessary and can be of some help.

The brain needs constant energy, consumes 20% of what the total body needs, and can't store any energy. The vital functions such as breathing, circulation, and organ functions must have its energy, and the complex cognitive functions will slow down.

We need to think about brain fatigue with curiosity and from a new perspective. It can otherwise be difficult to understand why ordinary fun and relaxing activities can be difficult to manage and consume disproportionately more energy for the person suffering from brain fatigue. Conversation for meaning with friends or reading a text in a newspaper or a book can take an enormous amount of energy. Usually, we think of this as relaxing. We also think of the coffee break at work as relaxing, but for a brain-fatigued person, this can be completely unbearable and takes a lot of energy. The result is that it is not a restful break, quite the opposite. To understand brain fatigue or the lack of energy that follows, we need to think in terms of brain activity, i.e., how energy-consuming it is regardless of activity. It is also important to understand the effect of all the impressions the brain is constantly exposed to, consciously as well as unconsciously. The person suffering from brain fatigue reports this as being overwhelming and can't filter out the redundant information. Letting the sound from the fan rest in the background, or the music in the restaurant, while talking to another person. It is all experienced and consumes energy.

The symptoms included in the Brain Fatigue Syndrome

Loss of energy

When suffering from brain fatigue, it leads to problems with work or stud ies as well as with private life. The mental energy quickly runs out; whatever you do, the more demanding the quicker. Sometimes, even a crippling exhaustion can strike very suddenly and unpredictably. The feeling is that all the energy is suddenly lost, and there is an urgent need for rest. Afterwards, it will take a disproportionately long time to regain the mental energy. It may seem that one should be able to sense it when the energy starts to wane, but it is most often very difficult to sense this and rest in time before it is too late. When symptoms are felt (central and associated) as headache, irritability, and not being able to follow the conversation, it is too late. It is thus problematic with the delayed experience and adaptation to the actual energy available.

> It is as if you squeeze out the last drop of energy there is and then there is no energy left. Then it is not possible to continue with anything. All that is needed is brain rest.

The result is that everyday activities can be very hard to manage, such as spending time with family and friends. This can be difficult for friends and family members to understand. Therefore, it can happen that friends try to give advice, according to what they experience as relaxing and helpful for well-being. They can say to the brain-fatigued person with well-meaning intention, "Let´s go out and meet some friends, you must have something else to think about that can cheer you up". But it doesn't work. It can be possible to stay for a short time if the place is calm, but this is hard to find if you go to a pub or restaurant.

Those suffering from brain fatigue are not lazy. Instead, they wish to be active, meet friends, and take part in society, more than what they have energy for. This is problematic, as social activities are important for emotional well-being.

Not being able to work or study is also extremely frustrating. Many people work full-time, collapse at home, and have hardly any energy left for anything else after a day's work. All the time at home must be devoted to resting to get through the next working day and the next working week. People report that if they have a partner, that person needs to take responsibility for most households, including children. In the long run, this is not durable, and it is a great risk that this results in total exhaustion and frustration. Part-time sick leave would, for a period, have been helpful. The whole life needs to be adapted to what energy exists.

Children also suffer from brain fatigue after illnesses or congenital diseases. It can be very difficult to manage school as well as cope with friends and leisure activities. There is a risk that teachers and parents with the best intentions push the child with too much extra help and support, but there must be a balance between activity and rest.

It is common from time to time to be completely exhausted. This applies above all at the beginning, before strategies and knowledge about how to manage the lack of energy exist. It's not harmful to exceed the limit and become completely depleted of energy occasionally, but it is not beneficial if this occurs often. Then brain fatigue can become even worse.

Long recovery time

The need for prolonged recovery is very characteristic of brain fatigue. After an effort that requires mental activation and attention, it takes a disproportionately long time, sometimes up to several days, to regain mental energy. A short break does not help if you are drained out of energy.

> The problem is that when you run out of energy, I am done for that day.

Difficult to concentrate and overwhelmed by impressions

Concentration difficulties are central in brain fatigue. There is a reduced ability to maintain attention for a longer period. Focus is easily lost. Conversations, especially with several people, are one of the tasks most difficult to manage and a great frustration. It is not only the content itself, what is said, communication is also gestures and mimics, and what is implied with the wording. All must be interpreted automatically and fast. When this doesn't work well, fast and efficiently, it will be difficult to follow the conversation, take an active part, and later remember what was discussed.

In addition, the person is easily distracted by whatever appears around, such as sounds, visual impressions, but also by their thoughts. The feeling of being overwhelmed with impressions is common, and linked to this is the inability to "filter" the redundant impression to the background. Normally, attention can be maintained for longer periods, and the sounds that are in the background disappear and do not take place in consciousness. For a brain-fatigued person, background noise and visual impressions compete. Maybe this is one of the reasons for being easily exhausted during mental activities. It will also be difficult to manage several activities simultaneously. There is a need to do one thing at a time and at a slower pace.

> When I get tired, I can't keep up with conversations. I lose track of what is being said. I cannot pick up nuances, gestures and what is said "between the lines". I can forget what to say and sometimes what I say is completely wrong. I really want to hang out with people and meet new and old friends. But because my brain gets tired so quickly, I don't meet people as often as I'd like.

There is often also a strong desire to spend time with family and friends and do things together, like going to the cinema or a football match. However, during all these activities, there are a lot of impressions, which take a large amount of energy for a brain-fatigued person.

Another common problem is that it is difficult to read a book, or texts in newspapers or on the computer. It can also be difficult to catch up on reading the subtitles on TV and in films. There is common reading slower and many stop reading books as it is not possible reading for meaning, and is also very tiresome. Following a film can also be hard, especially if many people are involved and there are many details to keep in order. There is a pace in society that we cannot control, and that becomes difficult to manage.

Brain fatigue varies

When the mental energy is reduced due to extensive mental work, it will take a long time to regain the energy lost. This results in difficulties, not only throughout the day, but also between days. Most people who suffer from brain fatigue report having more energy in the morning and worse in the afternoon and evening. If a lot of energy has been used one day, the next day may start at a slightly lower energy level compared to the day before, having less energy for daily activities, and it will not be possible to do as much as the day before. This also makes it problematic when trying to find a good balance between activities and rest, as it varies.

Memory problems

People who suffer from brain fatigue commonly report memory problems. For example, not remembering what was discussed during the conversation. It may not have to be a memory problem, but it can be an effect of attention not working well enough. A neuropsychological assessment can clarify this.

Slowness of thinking

Slowness of thinking is a common complaint. It can also be a slowness in other activities, such as reading.

Reduced initiative

Suffering from brain fatigue means that it can be very difficult to get started with activities, even with everyday tasks. For example, it can be difficult to deal with laundry and dishes, sort mail, and pay bills.

> The worst thing is that I feel lazy, because I can't manage it. But I simply can't do it.

Irritability and tearfulness

Many people get easily irritated, even for tiny things, and it passes away quickly. For many, it is also common to be more emotional and tearful than before. Both can be troublesome for the person himself and for people nearby.

Sleep problems

Many suffer from sleep disturbances and do not feel rested when woken up. It can be problems with difficulties falling asleep, fragmented sleep, sleeping more superficially, episodes with wakefulness, or sleeping much more than is normal. It can also happen that longer periods of more sleep alternate with periods of shorter sleep and poorer sleep quality. Following over-exertion, the sleep can become worse, and after a period of rest and calm, sleep can improve.

Sound and light sensitivity

Many people who suffer from brain fatigue have problems with sound/noise and light sensitivity. Both can be experienced as much stronger than normal. Driving past can create a sound that hurts, and a fan in the background can be hard to tolerate. The visual impression of the sun reflecting on the snow or on the water can be unbearable. Even strong indoor lighting can be difficult to manage.

Stress sensitivity

Most people with brain fatigue experience an increased sensitivity to stress. What could be managed without a problem before the injury or illness is experienced as more stressful. It can occur in situations where there is a lot of impression and a bit messy, and when demands are made to perform.

Headaches after mental activity

Headaches in the form of a pressing pain, sometimes with the feeling of a tightening band around the head are common, especially after exertion or too many impressions. It can take a while, maybe having a calm period after falling ill, but when it is time to be more active and resume work, the headache can be pronounced.

Bibliography

Andersen, G., Christensen, D., Kirkevold, M., & Johnsen, S. P. (2012). Post-stroke fatigue and return to work: A 2-year follow-up. *Acta Neurologica Scandinavica*, 125(4), 248–253. https://doi.org/10.1111/j.1600-0404.2011.01557.x. Epub 2011 Jun 21.

Cantor, J. B., Ashman, T., Gordon, W., Ginsberg, A., Engmann, C., Egan, M., . . . Flanagan, S. (2008). Fatigue after traumatic brain injury and its impact on participation and quality of life. *Journal of Head Trauma Rehabilitation*, 23(1), 41–51.

Eriksson, G., Larsson, I., Guidetti, S., & Johansson, U. (2023). Handling fatigue in everyday activities at five years after stroke: A long and demanding process. *Scandinavian Journal of Occupational Therapy*, February;30(2), 228–238. https://doi.org/10.1080/11038128.2022.2089230

Fahrenfort, J. J., Wilterdink, A. M. L., & van der Veen, E. A. (2000). Long-term residual complaints and psychosocial sequelae after remission of hyperthyroidism. *Psychoneuroendocrinology*, 25, 201–211.

Johansson, B. (2022). Screening method for assessment of work ability for patients suffering from mental fatigue front. *Behavioural Neuroscience*, 16, 869377. https://doi.org/10.3389/fnbeh.2022.869377

Johansson, B., Berglund, P., & Rönnbäck, L. (2009). Mental fatigue and impaired information processing after mild and moderate traumatic brain injury. *Brain Injury*, 23(13–14), 1027–1040.

Johansson, B., & Rönnbäck, L. (2025). The Brain Fatigue Syndrome—symptoms, probable definition, and pathophysiological mechanisms. *Journal of Clinical Medicine*, 14(3271). https://doi.org/10.3390/jcm 14103271

Norlander, A., Lindgren, I., Pessah-Rasmussen, H., Gard, G., & Brogårdh, C. (2021). Fatigue in men and women who have returned to work after stroke: Assessed with the fatigue severity scale and mental fatigue scale. *Journal of Rehabilitation Medicine*, 9, 53(jrm00227). https://doi.org/10.2340/16501977-2863

Raichle, M. E. (2015). The restless brain: How intrinsic activity organizes brain function. *Philosophical Transactions of the Royal Society*, 19;370(1668), 20140172. https://doi.org/10.1098/rstb.2014.0172

van de Port, I. G., Kwakkel, G., Schepers, V. P., Heinemans, C. T., & Lindeman, E. (2007). Is fatigue an independent factor associated with activities of daily living, instrumental activities of daily living and health-related quality of life in chronic stroke? *Cerebrovascular Diseases*, 23(1), 40–45.

3 Brain Fatigue Syndrome and pain

Individuals affected by Brain Fatigue Syndrome often experience persistent pain and discomfort. This pain may initially be triggered by an injury to a specific part of the body. However, it frequently becomes prolonged and chronic, and not uncommonly, it spreads to larger areas of the body. It is believed that the nerve cells responsible for sensing pain impulses become overactive, sending excessive pain signals to the brain, a phenomenon referred to as pain spread.

Importantly, this does not imply that the original site of injury has expanded or that the initial damage has worsened rather than healed, as one might expect. Instead, the brain may respond in a way that causes the individual to perceive the pain as more widespread or intense. This phenomenon is well documented, and affected individuals should not feel as though they are exaggerating or simulating their symptoms. For some, this is a genuine experience.

The underlying mechanisms remain unclear, but one hypothesis is that a dysfunction in signal transmission between brain cells may be involved, potentially due to an inflammatory condition. This could lead to the activation of microglia and astrocytes in the brain, initiating a vicious cycle of sustained neuroinflammation. Additionally, mast cells may play a significant role by contributing to the activation of other cells with inflammatory properties, thereby promoting inflammation within the nervous system.

While current understanding is still speculative, these mechanisms offer a plausible hypothetical explanation for the condition that affects many individuals.

DOI: 10.4324/9781003732105-3

Bibliography

Chen, Q., Bharadwaj, V., Irvine, K.-A., & Clark, J. D. (2023). Mechanisms and treatments of chronic pain after traumatic brain injury. *Neurochemistry International*, 19(171), 105630. https://doi.org/10.1016/j.neuint.2023.105630

Scholz, J. (2014). Mechanisms of chronic pain. *Molecular Pain*, 15;10(suppl 1), O15. https://doi.org/10.1186/1744-8069-10-S1-O15

Scholz, J., & Woolf, C. J. (2007). The neuropathic pain triad: Neurons, immune cells and glia. *Nature Neuroscience*, 10, 1361–1368. https://doi.org/10.1038/nn1992

4 Assessment of Brain Fatigue Syndrome

To provide the best possible treatment for Brain Fatigue Syndrome, a thorough investigation is essential. An in-depth analysis must always be conducted. This includes interviewing the patient about their medical history, previous illnesses, abilities, education, and work. When possible, relatives should also be included in the assessment. Social factors that may impact the condition need to be explored as well. Several factors may influence the severity of fatigue, including poor sleep, emotional disorders, medication, cognitive impairment, and other preexisting conditions.

Alternative diagnoses that could explain the fatigue must be investigated. These can include depression, anxiety, narcolepsy, neurological diseases, early signs of dementia, psychiatric and neuropsychiatric disorders such as autism and ADHD, and other somatic and endocrine dysfunctions. It is also important to explore developmental disorders from childhood and any injuries sustained early in life. Completing this puzzle is crucial for an accurate diagnosis.

> I've had brain fatigue for almost four years, which has gradually improved but is still far from good. It wasn't until now that I discovered by chance that it's brain fatigue I'm suffering from. Sometimes, I've been sure that I'm going crazy. For four years, I've seen several different doctors who have looked at me like a question mark when I describe my symptoms. Luckily, a few weeks ago, I found an article about brain fatigue, and everything fell into place. Since finding this, life has already gotten better, and I see new light. Until now, I thought I was alone in this condition, so this feels hopeful.

DOI: 10.4324/9781003732105-4

Recommended assessment of Brain Fatigue Syndrome

To provide the best possible treatment for Brain Fatigue Syndrome, a thorough investigation is essential. The following examinations may be considered to exclude other diagnoses and underlying problems:

1. Brain Imaging: Computer X-ray (CT) and/or MRI scans, as well as cerebral blood flow studies, typically show no specific changes related to brain fatigue. However, these should be carried out if clinical indications exist, such as ambiguity regarding the underlying causes of brain fatigue.
2. Blood Tests: A comprehensive blood count with basal samples, quick-sink (CRP), and regular lowering (SR) can reveal current infections. Additionally, monitoring blood sugar, blood fats (lipid status), thyroid function (TSH, free T3, and free T4), iron status (iron and ferritin), zinc, and vitamin D is important. The function of the parathyroid glands should also be examined with tests for parathyroid hormone (PTH), calcium (Ca^{2+}), and vitamin B-related substances (B12/cobalamin, folacin, and homocysteine). Homocysteine tests may indicate deficiencies in folic acid and vitamin B12.
3. Spinal Fluid Examination: This can rule out underlying infections or inflammations of the nervous system, such as TWAR, Lyme disease, mycoplasma, EBV, and CMV. TWAR is an insidious bronchial disease that can affect a person without their knowledge. Mononucleosis, caused by the Epstein–Barr virus (EBV), is a form of glandular fever. In previously healthy individuals, CMV infection usually produces no symptoms, while those with compromised immune systems can experience inflammation in several organs.
4. Consulting with an endocrinological expert is advisable if the cause of brain fatigue remains unclear.

It is also important to conduct neuropsychological and occupational assessments, as well as use assessment scales for fatigue.

Questionnaires for fatigue

Many rating scales exist to measure fatigue; up to 71 have been reported in research. Some scales assess fatigue in general, while others are multidimensional, distinguishing between physical, social, and mental fatigue, as well as specific activities related to fatigue. Certain scales are adapted for specific disorders, while others are recommended for broader populations. Different scales are used for children and adults.

Many scales use a numerical rating system, typically ranging from 0 (no problems) to 5 (severe problems). Alternatively, responses may be indicated on a line between two extremes, such as low to high fatigue. Some questionnaires, like the Mental Fatigue Scale (MFS) that we have used, offer predefined response options and assess multiple symptoms (see Appendix). The MFS has been evaluated for use in adults.

It is up to clinicians and researchers to choose the scale most appropriate for the specific situation. This approach is similar to assessments of depression, anxiety, or quality of life, where rating scales are often used when no better assessment tools are available.

Mental Fatigue Scale – The self-assessment scale for Brain Fatigue Syndrome

We have long used the self-rating Mental Fatigue Scale (MFS) in research and clinical settings. The MFS has been evaluated for people with acquired brain injuries and later used for various groups suffering from brain fatigue, such as those with cerebral palsy, endocrine disorders, multiple sclerosis, and burnout syndrome. The MFS encompasses a complex of symptoms commonly reported after neurological disorders, based on extensive clinical experience.

The MFS includes specific questions about general fatigue, mental fatigue related to mental activity, the extra need for recovery time after exhaustion, lack of initiative, cognitive complaints (such as concentration and memory problems), slowness of thinking, emotional problems (such as irritability and tearfulness), sensory sensitivity (to light and sound), stress sensitivity, and sleep problems. There is also an extra question about diurnal variation, addressing the impact of brain fatigue throughout the day (not included in the total sum of score). Despite the seemingly different symptoms, they are all closely related and have a high internal consistency. A value above 10 indicates significant problems with brain fatigue, with higher values indicating greater severity. The MFS has not been shown to be related to age (applies to ages 20–65), gender, or education. It is also possible to respond to MFS using a mobile application. The data will be stored on the personal mobile device and can help track personal changes over time in relation to activities performed. This could be useful for monitoring the effects of increasing or decreasing working hours. What will happen?

The MFS questions have predefined alternative answers, ensuring that everyone relates to the questions similarly. This consistency is important for reliable ratings over time. The construction is similar to the Beck Depression Inventory (BDI) and the Montgomery-Åsberg Depression

Rating Scale (MADRS) for assessing depression, which also use predefined alternatives. A drawback of predefined alternatives is that it can be tiresome or difficult to keep all information in mind while making decisions, so assistance from someone may be necessary.

The close relationship between specific questions from the MFS and how they change in synchrony is illustrated in Figure 4.1. This means that if Brain Fatigue Syndrome improves, concentration improves, noise sensitivity decreases, and irritability lessens, among other symptoms. The figure is based on a medical study with methylphenidate after a traumatic brain injury (TBI) (more about this study in the treatment section). The figure shows how every single question from the MFS is reported without treatment, with a low dose (15 mg/day), and a normal dose (60 mg/day) of methylphenidate. The highest ratings (most problems) are seen with no drug, intermediate ratings with a low dose, and the lowest ratings with a normal dose for all separate symptoms.

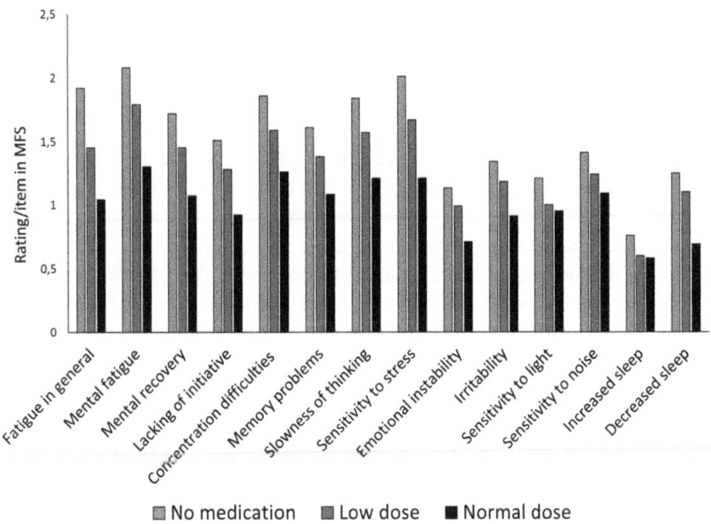

Figure 4.1 The figure shows how each individual item on the Mental Fatigue Scale (MFS) is rated under three conditions: without treatment, with a low dose (15 mg/day), and with a standard dose (60 mg/day) of methylphenidate. The highest symptom ratings (indicating the most severe problems) are found without medication, intermediate ratings with the low dose, and the lowest ratings with the standard dose across all symptoms. (The figure is from Johansson B, and Rönnbäck L. 2025. *J. Clin. Med.*, 14(3271). Doi:10.3390/jcm14103271).

Headache and brain fatigue

We have not included headaches in the MFS, but we are well aware that they commonly occur and are closely connected with mental activity and Brain Fatigue Syndrome. For many, headaches appear when life demands increase, such as returning to work after an illness. Headaches improve when activities are better adapted to the person's brain fatigue. It is important to understand the headache described by the patient and ask about when and how it occurs.

Is the self-assessment reliable?

The self-assessment scales for fatigue are the best tools we have today, similar to those used for assessing depression and anxiety. No objective biomarker exists, so we must rely on thorough assessments for brain fatigue. Our clinical experience shows that most patients answer accurately, reflecting their everyday activities. Occasionally, patients may underreport their symptoms due to severe memory problems or lack of awareness, especially in the early stages of rehabilitation. As patients gain knowledge and insight during rehabilitation, their MFS scores may increase as they better understand their condition. Severe memory problems can result in lower ratings, even when brain fatigue is evident to those around the patient. Overestimating problems is rare but can be clarified through discussions with the patient about the MFS questions and their daily life.

It is always important to discuss each MFS question and everyday life with the patient, providing valuable information for healthcare professionals and helping patients become more aware of their difficulties. Involving relatives can also help them better understand Brain Fatigue Syndrome.

In comparison, the MFS has a strong positive correlation with the Fatigue Severity Scale and the Fatigue Impact Scale (FIS) and is best for FIS subscale cognitive fatigue, intermediate for psychosocial fatigue, and less for physical fatigue.

One type of Brain Fatigue Syndrome?

We have used the MFS for various diagnostic groups over a long period, and it has become clear that Brain Fatigue Syndrome exists across many diagnostic groups. They report very similar symptoms and difficulties when brain fatigue is present.

Assessment by an occupational therapist

An occupational therapist can assess the affected person's daily and weekly activities to identify what they do and when, and whether there's enough time for rest. Often, people don't realize how much they actually accomplish and might think, "I haven't done anything today." However, a detailed investigation can reveal that a lot gets done, including routine tasks and even small chores. It's important to allocate time for personal care, meal preparation, and physical activities like walking. By creating a detailed overview of their day and week, they can see the balance between mental activities and rest. This might highlight the need for changes. Understanding which activities drain their energy and which ones are restful is crucial for developing strategies to achieve a more balanced daily life.

Cognitive assessment by a neuropsychologist

Investigating cognitive function often requires a neuropsychological examination. Cognitive impairments can add extra burdens, particularly in the acute phase. Recognizing and understanding these impairments is essential, and rehabilitation must be tailored to address them as well as Brain Fatigue Syndrome. It's also important to identify cognitive functions that remain intact and inform the person about that. People often worry about memory problems and their reduced cognitive efficiency. They need to understand their cognitive abilities and how they relate to Brain Fatigue Syndrome.

In research studies, the mean values for neuropsychological tests for those with Brain Fatigue Syndrome after a brain injury often show reduced processing speed and attention on the group level compared to healthy control participants. However, in the clinical setting, many who suffer from Brain Fatigue Syndrome report severe cognitive difficulties in everyday life, yet they often perform within the normal range on cognitive tests. However, neuropsychological tests are designed to identify focal brain damage and are not aimed at predicting everyday function. The discrepancy between objective cognitive function and subjective cognitive complaints can be confusing for patients. This discrepancy has been observed in patients with burnout syndrome (BOS) and Graves' disease (hyperthyroidism) compared to controls. Our studies show a similar pattern, as illustrated in Figure 4.2, for participants reporting brain fatigue after a TBI or BOS. Z-value normalizes different raw scores to a common value, making it possible to compare different tests and scores from the MFS with equal values. The figure shows that subjectively reported cognitive problems in MFS (concentration, memory, slowness of thinking) are more pronounced, while differences in cognitive test results are minimal compared to controls (tests include processing speed as digit symbol coding, and working memory, both from WAIS).

Cognitive tests can yield perfect results, but if we don't consider what happens afterward, we miss crucial information. Total exhaustion for days can follow a neuropsychological assessment, even when the test

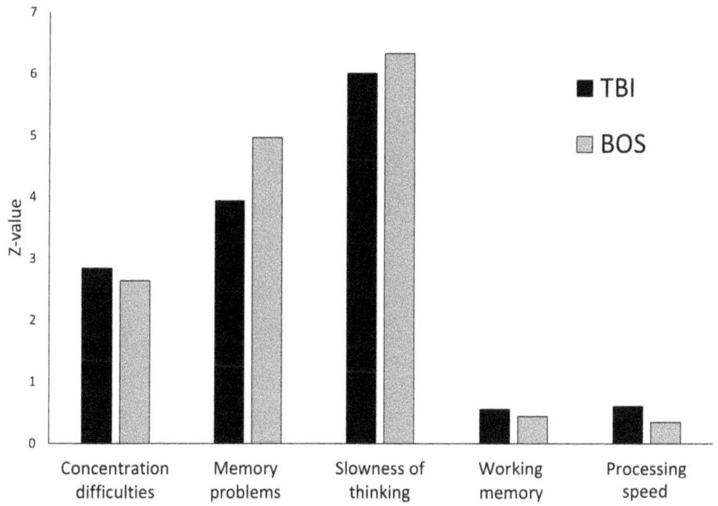

Figure 4.2 Comparison of Z-values for subjective cognitive complaints, based on items from the Mental Fatigue Scale (MFS), including concentration, memory, and slowness of thinking, and objective cognitive tests (digit span for working memory, digit symbol coding for processing speed), in individuals with traumatic brain injury (TBI) and burnout syndrome (BOS).

situation adheres to ethical principles. Endurance is essential in everyday life, yet traditional neuropsychological tests do not account for it. For those suffering from brain fatigue, there's a significant discrepancy between their performance on cognitive tests and their ability to sustain mental tasks and maintain work or mental activities throughout the day without experiencing total exhaustion.

Bibliography

Anderson, J. F. I., & Cockle, E. (2021). Investigating the effect of fatigue and psychological distress on information processing speed in the postacute period after mild traumatic brain injury in premorbidly healthy adults. *Archives of Clinical Neuropsychology*, 4, acaa123. https://doi.org/10.1093/arclin/acaa123

Andreasen, A. K., Spliid, P. E., Andersen, H., & Jakobsen, J. (2010). Fatigue and processing speed are related in multiple sclerosis. *European Journal of Neurology*, 17(2), 212–218. https://doi.org/10.1111/j.1468-1331.2009.02776.x

Ashman, T. A., Cantor, J. B., Gordon, W. A., Spielman, L., Egan, M., Ginsberg, A., . . . Flanagan, S. (2008). Objective measurement of fatigue following traumatic brain injury. *Journal of Head Trauma Rehabilitation*, 23(1), 33–40.

Hjollund, N. H., Andersen, J. H., & Bech, P. (2007). Assessment of fatigue in chronic disease: A bibliographic study of fatigue measurement scales. *Health and Quality of Life Outcomes*, 27(5), 12. https://doi.org/10.1186/1477-7525-5-12

Johansson, B., Berglund, P., & Rönnbäck, L. (2009). Mental fatigue and impaired information processing after mild and moderate traumatic brain injury. *Brain Injury*, 23(13–14), 1027–1040.

Johansson, B., Holmberg, M., Skau, S., Malmgren, H., & Filipsson Nyström, H. (2023). The relationship between mental fatigue, depression, and cognition in Graves' disease. *European Thyroid Journal*, 12(4), e230040. https://doi.org/10.1530/ETJ-23-0040

Johansson, B., & Rönnbäck, L. (2012). Mental fatigue and cognitive impairment after an almost neurological recovered stroke. *International Scholarly Research Network Psychiatry*, 2012(Article ID 686425), 7. https://doi.org/10.5402/2012/686425

Johansson, B., & Rönnbäck, L. (2014). Evaluation of the mental fatigue scale and its relation to cognitive and emotional functioning after traumatic brain injury or stroke. *International Journal of Physical Medicine and Rehabilitation*, 2, 182. https://doi.org/10.4172/2329-9096.1000182

Johansson, B., & Rönnbäck, L. (2025). The Brain Fatigue Syndrome—Symptoms, probable definition, and pathophysiological mechanisms. *Journal of Clinical Medicine*, 14(3271). https://doi.org/10.3390/jcm14103271

Johansson, B., Wentzel, A.-P., Andréll, P., Mannheimer, C., & Rönnbäck, L. (2015). Methylphenidate reduces mental fatigue and improves processing speed in persons suffered a traumatic brain injury. *Brain Injury*, 29(6), 758–765.

Möller, M. C., Nygren de Boussard, C., Oldenburg, C., & Bartfai, A. (2014). An investigation of attention, executive, and psychomotor aspects of cognitive fatigability. *Journal of Clinical and Experimental Neuropsychology*, 36(7), 716–729

Nelson, A., Malmberg Gavelin, H., Boraxbekk, C.-J., Eskilsson, T., Josefsson, M., Slunga Järvholm, L., & Stigsdotter Neely, A. (2021). Subjective cognitive complaints in patients with stress-related exhaustion disorder: A cross sectional study. *BMC Psychology*, 9(1), 84. https://doi.org/10.1186/s40359-021-00576-9

Skau, S., Bunketorp-Käll, L., Kuhn, H. G., & Johansson, B. (2019). Mental fatigue and functional near-infrared spectroscopy (fNIRS) – Based assessment of cognitive performance after mild traumatic brain injury. *Frontiers Human Neuroscience*, 13(145). https://doi.org/10.3389/fnhum.2019.00145

Skau, S., Jonsdottir, I. H., Sjörs Dahlman, A., Johansson, B., & Kuhn, H. G. (2021). Exhaustion disorder and altered brain activity in frontal cortex detected with fNIRS. *Stress and Health*, 24(1), 64–75. https://doi.org/10.1080/10253890.2020.1777972

Wechsler, D. (2010). *Wechsler Adult Intelligence Scale*, 3rd ed., WAIS-IV, Swedish version. Pearson Assessment.

Ziino, C., & Ponsford, J. (2006). Selective attention deficits and subjective fatigue following traumatic brain injury. *Neuropsychology*, 20, 383–390.

5 Depression and anxiety

When someone suffers an acquired brain injury or is diagnosed with a neurological disease, depression and anxiety can develop. Depression and anxiety can also be a consequence of Brain Fatigue Syndrome.

Depression and anxiety correlate with brain fatigue and can coexist. However, brain fatigue after a traumatic brain injury (TBI) is suggested to be related to the brain injury itself, rather than as a consequence of anxiety and depression. For instance, brain fatigue did not improve with the antidepressant fluoxetine after a brain injury. Fatigue also uniquely contributes to disability after TBI, even when controlling for injury severity, executive functions, and depression status. Brain fatigue is also a distinct state in endocrine conditions like Graves' disease and can exist without depression.

Differentiating between Brain Fatigue Syndrome and depression can be challenging due to symptom overlaps in questionnaires, such as concentration problems, reduced initiative, irritability, and sleep disturbances. However, both Brain Fatigue Syndrome and depression can occur together.

In depression, central symptoms include a depressed mood most of the day, diminished interest or pleasure in activities, inability to feel joy, pessimism, reduced zest for life, changes in sleeping patterns, and fatigue. The distinguishing feature of Brain Fatigue Syndrome is that the person has the will to do things, has an interest, and wants to be active. They often try to do more than what is appropriate, leading to exhaustion and a need for long mental recovery. It is also typical to have a clear variation in symptoms throughout the day and between days for those suffering from Brain Fatigue Syndrome. Additionally, these individuals are clearly affected by the activities they perform and are not apathetic or lazy.

Different treatments are considered for depression and anxiety, and must be managed in relation to brain fatigue. Briefly, depression can be treated with antidepressant medication, psychotherapy, or a combination of both. This also applies to anxiety. If Brain Fatigue Syndrome coexists with depression and/or anxiety, the treatment must be chosen with awareness and adapted to the person's brain fatigue. Emotional instability and

DOI: 10.4324/9781003732105-5

irritability are significant symptoms related to brain fatigue and can be alleviated with a low dose of antidepressants, although this does not improve the fatigue itself.

In summary, depression, anxiety, and brain fatigue need to be regarded as separate states.

Bibliography

Choi-Kwon, S., Choi, J., Kwon, S. U., Kang, D.-W., & Kim, J. S. (2007). Fluoxetine is not effective in the treatment of post-stroke fatigue: A double-blind, placebo-controlled study. *Cerebrovascular Diseases*, 23(2–3), 103–108. https://doi.org/10.1159/000097045

Johansson, B., Berglund, P., & Rönnbäck, L. (2009). Mental fatigue and impaired information processing after mild and moderate traumatic brain injury. *Brain Injury*, 23(13–14), 1027–1040.

Johansson, B., Holmberg, M., Skau, S., Malmgren, H., & Filipsson Nyström, H. (2023). The relationship between mental fatigue, depression, and cognition in Graves' disease. *European Thyroid Journal*, 12(4), e230040. https://doi.org/10.1530/ETJ-23-0040

Johansson, B., & Rönnbäck, L. (2012). Mental fatigue and cognitive impairment after an almost neurological recovered stroke. *International Scholarly Research Network Psychiatry*, 2012(Article ID 686425), 7. https://doi.org/10.5402/2012/686425

Juengst, S., Skidmore, E., Arenth, P. M., Niyonkuru, C., & Raina, K. D. (2013). The unique contribution of fatigue to disability in community dwelling adults with traumatic brain injury. *Archives of Physical Medicine and Rehabilitation*, 94(1), 74–79.

Ponsford, J., Schönberger, M., & Rajaratnam, S. M. W. (2015). A model of fatigue following traumatic brain injury. *Journal of Head Trauma Rehabilitation*, 20(4), 277–283. https://doi.org/10.1097/HTR.0000000000000049

Staub, F., & Bogousslavsky, J. (2001). Fatigue after stroke: A major but neglected issue. *Cerebrovascular Diseases*, 12, 75–81.

6 Probable pathophysiology of Brain Fatigue Syndrome at the cellular level

There is no proof today that any specific brain area is more susceptible to the development of brain fatigue. Furthermore, there is no connection between the severity of the brain injury and brain fatigue. Brain fatigue can occur with any disease affecting the brain, not for all, and its magnitude is personal.

While we still don't fully understand how the brain works, and likely only know a fraction of its neurotransmitters and signalling systems, it's clear that the brain strives to operate with high energy efficiency, specificity, and speed. This efficiency likely explains our ability to quickly identify and process incoming information, integrating it with existing knowledge and emotional responses. The brain functions as a cohesive unit, meaning all areas and signalling systems must be intact for optimal performance.

Processes like attention, concentration, information intake, and memory storage (cognition) are incredibly energy intensive. They require precise and rapid nerve cell signalling. Typically, information intake and processing are intertwined with emotional responses, leading to significant brain activity even during rest. During cognitive tasks, the demands for identifying and processing information increase, necessitating high specificity and speed, and thus, significant energy consumption. This means the brain must quickly integrate and store large amounts of information, comparing it with existing data with high precision and speed.

We are constantly bombarded with various stimuli: sound, light, taste, smell, and joint position. Normally, our brain's filter functions slow down unnecessary signals, preventing them from overwhelming the brain's identification and processing centres.

Many people with Brain Fatigue Syndrome experience a "foggy" feeling and sluggish thinking, possibly due to reduced mental and cognitive ability. When they exert cognitive effort, this sluggishness becomes more apparent. In our research, participants with brain fatigue from traumatic

DOI: 10.4324/9781003732105-6

head injuries reported that methylphenidate, which increases dopamine and norepinephrine in the brain's frontal regions, made them feel more "clear-headed" and "alert." However, they generally lacked the energy to increase their work capacity.

Additionally, Brain Fatigue Syndrome sufferers are inundated with impressions, some of which are trivial, due to impaired filter functions. This overloads the brain's centres for identifying and processing information. While the nerve cells and networks do not function correctly, greater resources are needed for cognitive activities. This may be due to more non-specific glutamate signalling (more noise in synaptic transmission) and the engagement of larger neuronal networks in cognitive processes in Brain Fatigue Syndrome.

Brain imaging and fatigue

Brain imaging studies on fatigue are limited and vary in design, but they have reported notable changes. Using functional near-infrared spectroscopy (fNIRS), we observed that from the start of the experiment, individuals with brain fatigue showed lower frontal cortex activity (lower peak oxygenated haemoglobin in response to a task) compared to healthy controls during cognitive tests. Those suffering from brain fatigue due to traumatic brain injury or burnout syndrome reported increased fatigue after two and a half hours of mental activity, unlike the controls. However, their brain activity levels were lower from the beginning and remained unchanged over the 2.5-hour period. Similarly, functional magnetic resonance imaging (fMRI) revealed lower brain activity in the TBI group compared to controls. While controls showed decreased brain activity over a 27-minute test session, the TBI group maintained consistently lower brain activity levels. Other researchers have also reported altered brain activation and connectivity in relation to fatigue in TBI patients. These findings suggest that brain function differs significantly when brain fatigue is present.

Probable pathophysiology of Brain Fatigue Syndrome at the cellular level

Brain fatigue appears to result from a combination of neurobiological dysfunctions, including impaired neurotransmission, neuroinflammation, reduced cerebral energy supply, and inefficient neural network activation. In individuals with brain fatigue, larger and more energy-demanding neuronal networks may be recruited for cognitive processing, reflecting a compensatory but inefficient mechanism.

Several hypotheses have been proposed to explain the underlying mechanisms of brain fatigue:

- Dopamine Imbalance Hypothesis
- Serotonin Hypothesis
- Acetylcholine Hypothesis
- Cytokine Hypothesis
- Mitochondrial Dysfunction Hypothesis
- Astroglial–Glutamate Dysfunction Hypothesis

Although direct dysfunction in a specific neurotransmitter system has not been conclusively identified, dysregulation of neurotransmitters, particularly dopamine, serotonin, and norepinephrine is likely to play central roles.

Dopamine levels have been shown to decline during sustained cognitive activity, and this reduction correlates with subjective experiences of mental exhaustion. However, dopamine dysfunction alone cannot fully account for brain fatigue. For example, in our studies, administration of methylphenidate, which increases dopamine and norepinephrine levels in the frontal cortex, does not alleviate all symptoms associated with Brain Fatigue Syndrome.

Serotonin and norepinephrine levels are also affected during brain fatigue. Serotonin dysregulation is thought to contribute to fatigue in conditions such as depression and chronic fatigue syndrome.

Acetylcholine, essential for cognitive alertness, may also be involved. Additionally, the accumulation of metabolic by-products such as adenosine may exacerbate fatigue. Adenosine inhibits neural activity and accumulates during prolonged mental exertion. Sleep, which facilitates the clearance of metabolic waste products, can temporarily alleviate brain fatigue.

In inflammatory diseases such as multiple sclerosis, brain fatigue is common and appears to be independent of disease activity or demyelination. Disturbed dopamine signalling involving the basal ganglia, thalamus, and frontal lobes has been proposed. While these regions are implicated, brain fatigue can arise from dysfunction in various brain areas.

This suggests that Brain Fatigue Syndrome may involve a multifactorial mechanism, including disrupted neurotransmitter homeostasis and impaired cerebral energy metabolism. The brain may compensate by activating broader, less efficient neuronal systems. Such nonspecific activation deviates from the brain's typical energy-efficient signalling patterns. This hypothesis aligns with findings from traumatic brain injury research, where brain fatigue is associated with compensatory neural activity due to disrupted networks. Diffusion tensor imaging has revealed microstructural damage in white matter tracts, particularly in the corpus callosum and frontal lobes, which are critical for cognitive function. Neural network dysfunction may exacerbate brain fatigue.

Neuroinflammation may be a unifying factor. Disruption of extracellular homeostasis activates microglia, leading to the release of inflammatory mediators. Astrocytes respond by becoming reactive, altering their normal functions. Their ability to regulate synaptic glutamate transmission diminishes, resulting in reduced glucose uptake from the bloodstream.

Glucose is the brain's primary energy source. Impaired glucose transport into the brain can lead to cognitive deficits and fatigue. Functional MRI and PET studies have demonstrated reduced cerebral glucose metabolism in fatigued individuals, particularly in the frontal and parietal lobes.

Furthermore, glutamine production and protein synthesis decline, while extracellular glutamate levels slightly increase, causing membrane depolarization and a general reduction in synaptic transmission. Inter-astrocytic communication also shifts from calcium signalling to extracellular ATP signalling. ATP, beyond its role as an energy carrier, acts as a signalling molecule. Both microglia and astrocytes possess purinergic receptors that detect ATP, triggering the release of inflammatory substances. This may lead to sustained and amplified neuroinflammation.

We propose that brain fatigue may result from impaired glutamate signalling in the brain, characterized by reduced specificity and speed in glutamate transmission and a decreased supply of energy substrates to astroglial cells from the blood. This hypothesis stems from the central role of cognitive dysfunction in pathological fatigue and the crucial importance of glutamate transmission for cognitive processes like information processing and memory storage. We now extend our hypothesis to encompass all symptoms of Brain Fatigue Syndrome and link the proposed biochemical mechanisms to these symptoms.

Neurotransmitters in relation to Brain Fatigue Syndrome

Glutamate, an excitatory neurotransmitter in the central nervous system, plays a vital role in learning, memory, and mood regulation. Glutamate levels in the prefrontal cortex have also been suggested as a marker of brain fatigue. Gamma-aminobutyric acid (GABA), an important inhibitory transmitter, is involved in cognitive impairments and may play a role in information suppression. Dopamine selectively inhibits (GABA neurones) or enhances (glutamate neurones) synaptic signalling, supporting action, attention, motivation, and affect, and balances neural activity. Dopamine is essential for working memory, attention, and cognitive control. Norepinephrine regulates a wide range of cognitive functions, including working memory, learning, attention, memory consolidation and retrieval, vigilance, and wakefulness. The dorsolateral prefrontal cortex (DPFC) is sensitive to levels of norepinephrine and dopamine; norepinephrine is suggested to strengthen DPFC network connectivity, while dopamine decreases noise. Acetylcholine is another neurotransmitter important for attention, learning, and memory, enhancing the signal-to-noise ratio. Serotonin regulates mood, sleep, and cognition. After experimental brain injury, a long-term downregulation of glutamate, GABA, acetylcholine, norepinephrine, dopamine, and serotonin was reported. Although brain fatigue was not specifically addressed in that report, brain injuries commonly result in lasting Brain Fatigue Syndrome in humans, and these neurotransmitters are involved in cognitive, sensory, and emotional functions. Here, we discuss the connection between neurobiology and Brain Fatigue Syndrome and propose a model for this relationship.

Glutamate transmission

Glutamate is the most abundant excitatory neurotransmitter in the brain. It is stored in synaptic vesicles of nerve terminals until released. After interacting with glutamate receptors on the postsynaptic membrane, excess glutamate is cleared from the synaptic cleft by astroglial cells, enabling new, high-precision glutamate signalling with a high signal-to-noise ratio. In astrocytes, glutamate can be metabolized via the tricarboxylic acid cycle for protein synthesis or converted to glutamine and transferred back to the neuron. Astrocytes, along with neurones, are key players in glutamate transmission. They form large cell networks with long processes that enclose glutamate synapses and contact the walls of small blood vessels, together with endothelial cells, forming part of the blood-brain barrier (BBB). In addition to regulating ion and substance homeostasis in the extracellular environment, astrocytes are responsible for supplying energy to nerve cells and synapses.

Astrocytes: Star-shaped glial cells in the brain

- Most abundant cell type: Astrocytes are the most numerous cells in the brain.
- Complex structures: These cells have many long processes.
- Communication networks: Astrocytes communicate with each other through gap junctions, forming extensive three-dimensional networks.
- Multiple contacts: Their processes connect with synapses, nerve cell bodies, and brain cavities.
- Blood-Brain Barrier builders: They help construct parts of the blood-brain barrier (BBB).
- Immune activation: Astrocytes play a role in the brain's immune response.
- Homeostasis maintenance: They regulate the balance of ions and other substances in the extracellular fluid.
- Glutamate regulation: Astrocytes manage glutamate levels in the brain.

- Glucose uptake: They absorb glucose from the blood.
- Energy providers: Astrocytes supply energy substrates to nerve cells.

Microglial cells: The brain's immune defenders

- Immune surveillance: Microglial cells detect substances in the extracellular fluid.

Nerve cells: The brain's information relays

- Signal transmission: Nerve cells relay information through synaptic transmission.

Energy for the brain

Glucose is the brain's primary energy source, and a constant supply is essential for normal function. Synaptic transmission is highly energy-intensive, making the brain sensitive to glucose supply disruptions. Glucose metabolism in the brain can be studied using positron emission tomography (FDG-PET). Sustained brain hypometabolism or reduced glucose uptake has been observed days to months after a traumatic brain injury (TBI), though these results haven't been directly correlated with fatigue levels, and fatigue is a common long-term issue after TBI. FDG-PET studies have linked fatigue in Parkinson's disease to depressed metabolism in brain areas crucial for cognition and emotion, suggesting metabolic abnormalities and impaired functional interactions between brain regions. Similarly, glucose metabolism is significantly lower in multiple sclerosis (MS) and is thought to be linked to fatigue. Reduced or altered neuronal activation in response to cognitive activity has also been demonstrated.

Astrocytes primarily gain energy through glycolysis, while neurones rely on mitochondrial oxidative metabolism. Neuronal energy use is related to ion pump activity, which is crucial for establishing electrical gradients necessary for efficient neuronal activation and information transfer. Astrocytes are key in coupling synaptic activity with energy metabolism, transferring lactate to neurones. Both astrocytes and neurones increase their metabolic activity in response to heightened neurotransmission, a process regulated by glutamate signalling. For precise synaptic transmission, glutamate must be swiftly removed from the synaptic cleft, a task performed by astrocytes. These cells clear glutamate from the synaptic region once signalling is complete, ensuring low residual glutamate levels for continued high-precision signalling.

When astrocytes take up glutamate, they activate glucose uptake from the blood to provide energy for themselves, neurones, and synapses.

Glutamate taken up by astrocytes is converted into glutamine and transported back to nerve cells for the synthesis of new glutamate in excitatory neurones or GABA in inhibitory neurones. Glucose is not only an energy source but also a precursor for neurotransmitters like acetylcholine, glutamate, and GABA, as well as neuromodulators.

Impaired glutamate uptake by astrocytes

Studies have shown that astrocytes become inflamed during brain damage, affecting their communication and function. Inflammatory-activated astrocytes often lose their ability to effectively clear glutamate from synaptic clefts, leaving excess glutamate behind. This leads to imprecise glutamate signalling and non-specific activation of nerve cells due to excess glutamate in the extracellular space (Figure 6.1). Reduced glutamate uptake by astrocytes also results in lower protein formation and decreased production of other neurotransmitters, as well as reduced glucose uptake from the blood.

When glutamate uptake is impaired, extracellular glutamate levels rise, potentially leading to excitotoxicity. Even slightly elevated glutamate levels can cause non-specific activation of nearby neurones, activating larger cell networks in an uncoordinated manner. Additionally, astrocytes swell in response to increased extracellular glutamate, reducing their membrane

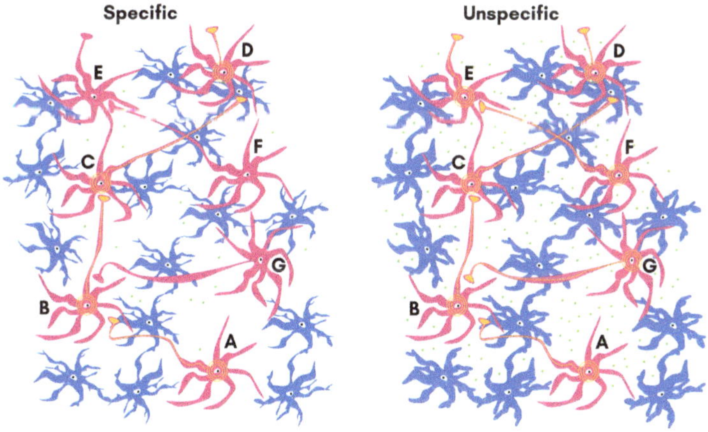

Figure 6.1 Specific activation (indicated in yellow within the pink neurones), illustrated in the left figure, is essential for fast and precise information processing. In this case, only neuron D is activated. The astrocytes (blue) regulate glutamate levels (green dots), returning them to a normal state and preparing the neuron for timely activation.

potential and capacity for potassium buffering. This creates a chaotic cellular environment where specific and non-specific signals are mixed.

Non-specific activation, illustrated in the right figure, occurs when inflammatory-activated astrocytes (blue and swollen) lose their ability to effectively clear glutamate from the synaptic clefts. This results in excess glutamate in the extracellular space (more green dots), leading to imprecise glutamate signalling (indicated in yellow) and non-specific activation of nerve cells, with both neurones E (non-specific) and D (specific) being activated.

The Brain Fatigue Syndrome and its relation to glutamate signalling

Reduced glutamate uptake by astrocytes may decrease glucose absorption from the blood, lowering energy availability in synapses, particularly those involved in higher brain functions like cognition and emotional responses. This reduced glutamate level interacts with dopamine, noradrenaline, serotonin (5-HT), acetylcholine, and GABA, all of which are suggested to be reduced in the chronic phase after a brain injury and are involved in many brain-related diseases. Supporting this, emotional symptoms can be alleviated by low-dose antidepressants, and attention problems can be relieved by medications like methylphenidate, which increases dopamine and noradrenaline in the synaptic space in frontal brain regions. Reduced GABA might be crucial for information filtering in the brain, and a decrease in GABA suppression of excitatory neural responses may lead to an overwhelming experience of impressions. If our hypothesis regarding the possible mechanisms of Brain Fatigue Syndrome at the cellular level is correct, we can expect that individuals with Brain Fatigue Syndrome have reduced glutamate uptake in astrocytes even at rest. Consequently, it is reasonable to imagine that these individuals have slightly elevated glutamate levels in the brain's extracellular fluid. A small amount of glutamate may diffuse into the extracellular space outside the synapses and activate other neurones non-specifically. However, this does not necessarily mean that extracellular glutamate levels reach excitotoxic levels, which can lead to nerve cell death. Instead, synaptic signalling becomes more imprecise with more "noise," as the synaptic cleft is not cleared of glutamate after signalling. This results in the activation of larger nerve cell and astrocyte networks, some of which are completely non-specific.

Slightly elevated extracellular glutamate levels also cause slight swelling of astrocytes and a decrease in the membrane potential of cell membranes. As astrocytes maintain the extracellular ion balance, including potassium (K^+), the K^+ content in the extracellular fluid may increase slightly due to the reduced membrane potential. This, in turn, means that synaptic neuronal signalling can be reduced not only for glutamate but probably for several transmitters. If our hypothesis is correct, this is a cellular starting point for Brain Fatigue Syndrome sufferers.

When a Brain Fatigue Syndrome sufferer engages in cognitive activity, impaired glutamate uptake in astrocytes may lead to further elevated glutamate levels in the synaptic cleft and extracellular space. This increases noise in glutamate signalling, reduces glutamate in astrocytes, decreases glutamine, and lowers glutamate in the tricarboxylic acid cycle for energy production. Additionally, glucose uptake by astrocytes from the blood decreases. The overall result may be the activation of larger brain areas with more widespread cell networks, some of which are completely non-specific, while the relative energy supply decreases. This may explain why Brain Fatigue Syndrome sufferers suddenly feel totally exhausted and completely "lost."

We should also consider that nerve cell signalling is likely to decrease in other transmitter systems as well, which may explain the associated symptoms of Brain Fatigue Syndrome.

How does this align with later findings that astrocytes can release a small amount of glutamate into the extracellular space? It has been speculated that this process, known as gliotransmission, is important for the excitability of nerve cells, likely helping them function optimally in both excitation and inhibition. We currently know too little about gliotransmission to fully understand and explain its significance in relation to Brain Fatigue Syndrome.

Long-term Brain Fatigue Syndrome

We know that most people recover from a mild TBI within one to three months, but others suffer from long-term fatigue. Thus, a mild injury may be anything but mild. For instance, 23% of individuals did not recover within a year after a mild TBI. Another study found that 30% had long-term problems, and a review indicated that approximately half of the individuals with a single mild TBI demonstrated long-term impairment. Worse outcomes can develop after recurrent mild TBIs. If brain fatigue persists for a year, there is a high risk that it will become a long-term or even chronic issue. The same scenario is observed after a minor stroke, indicating that the severity of the acquired brain injury does not predict long-term problems. Our studies have found lasting mental fatigue even five years after a TBI.

Since the extent of brain damage, location, age, or sex does not seem to influence the risk of long-lasting brain fatigue, one might wonder if there are pre-existing risk factors. Several studies suggest that individuals who suffer from depression and anxiety before the injury are more likely to experience long-term problems afterward. Pre-existing issues often become more pronounced and bothersome after an illness or injury. Genetic factors also play a role. People with a particular gene set of the apolipoprotein epsilon 4 allele are at greater risk of developing long-term brain fatigue after a brain injury.

How can this be? One probable explanation is that some individuals have different types of signalling between brain cells even before the injury or disease. In recent years, adenosine triphosphate (ATP) has been identified as a signalling molecule. Known as an energy substance, ATP has been shown to activate damaged cells not only in the brain but throughout the body.

In cases of brain damage resulting in neuroinflammation, it is now known that communication between astrocytes across gap junctions is closed and replaced by extracellular ATP signalling. Interestingly, microglial cells and astrocytes have receptors for ATP on their cell membranes and respond by forming and releasing inflammatory substances, including cytokines. These substances maintain the inflammatory status of astrocytes, reducing glutamate uptake and other properties. This creates a self-regulating cycle where inflammatory astrocytes persist. If our cellular model of Brain Fatigue Syndrome is correct, this may explain why Brain Fatigue Syndrome can be long-lasting.

Astrocytes may remain inflammatory-reactive with disturbed intercellular Ca^{2+} signalling and impaired glutamate uptake capacity. The gap junctions are closed, and the cells may have extracellular ATP signalling, stimulating purinergic receptors in microglia and astrocytes with the production of pro-inflammatory cytokines, and thus forming a self-maintaining circle where the astrocytes remain in an inflammatory reactive state (Figure 6.2).

Trauma or disease in the nervous system triggers neuroinflammation. This causes astrocytes to become inflammatory-reactive, reducing their ability to uptake glutamate and buffer potassium (K^+). As a result, extracellular levels of glutamate and K^+ slightly increase. The astrocytes swell slightly, and their membrane potential decreases due to the elevated extracellular K^+ levels. This reduction in membrane potential also affects neurones, potentially leading to decreased synaptic transmission.

The slight increase in extracellular glutamate causes more non-specific signalling, activating larger cell networks, some of which are non-specific. Reduced glutamate uptake by astrocytes leads to lower glutamate levels within these cells, resulting in less glutamine formation and potentially reduced glucose transport to the astrocytes. This results in an energy-deficient brain network and perception of brain fatigue.

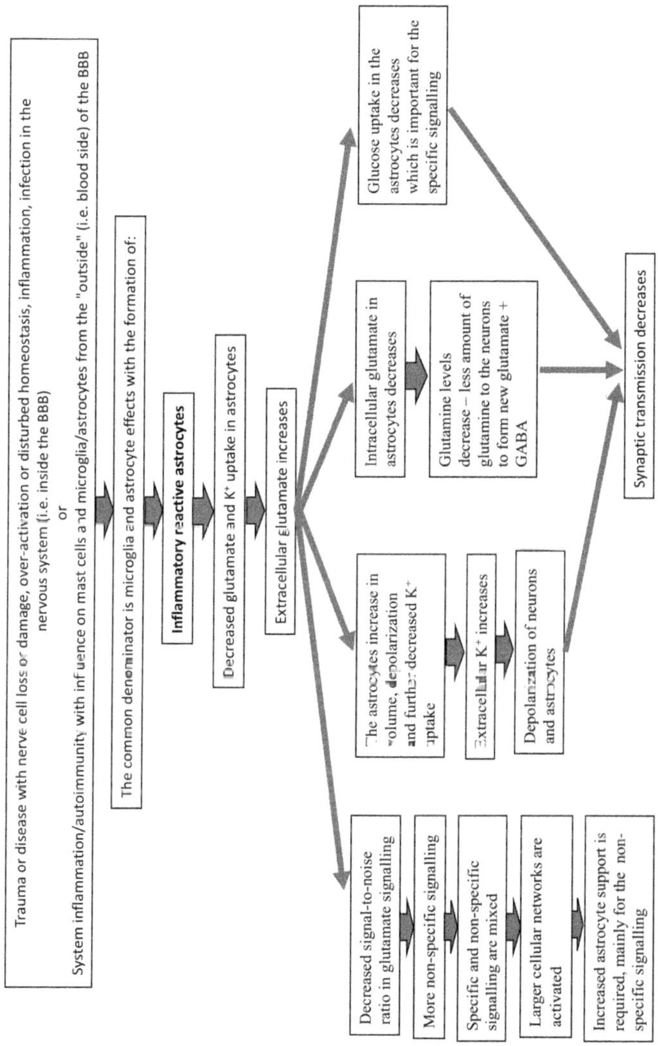

Figure 6.2 Schematic drawing of probable cellular events underlying Brain Fatigue Syndrome. (The figure is from Johansson B, and Rönnbäck L. 2025. *J. Clin. Med.*, 14(3271). Doi:10.3390/jcm14103271).

Bibliography

Abbott, N. J., Rönnbäck, L., & Hansson, E. (2006). Astrocyte-endothelial interactions at the blood-brain barrier. *Nature Reviews Neuroscience*, 7, 41–53.

Andersen, J. V. (2025). The glutamate/GABA- glutamine cycle: Insights, updates, and advances. *Journal of Neurochemistry*, 169, e70029. https://doi.org/10.1111/jnc.70029

Arnsten, A. F. T., & Dudley, A. G. (2005). Methylphenidate improves prefrontal cortical cognitive function through α2 adrenoceptor and dopamine D1 receptor actions: Relevance to therapeutic effects in attention deficit hyperactivity disorder. *Behavioral and Brain Functions*, April 22. https://doi.org/10.1186/1744-9081-1-2

Arnsten, A. R. T. (2011). Catecholamine influences on dorsolateral prefrontal cortical networks. *Biological Psychiatry*, 15(69), e89–99. https://doi.org/10.1016/j.biopsych.2011.01.027

Berginström, N., Nordström, P., Ekman, U., Eriksson, J., Andersson, M., Nyberg, L., & Nordström, A. (2018). Using functional magnetic resonance imaging to detect chronic fatigue in patients with previous traumatic brain injury: Changes linked to altered striato-thalamic-cortical functioning. *Journal of Head Trauma Rehabilitation*, 33(4), 266–274.

Byrnes, K. R., Wilson, C. M., Brabazon, F., von Leden, R., Jurgens, J. S., Oakes, T. R., & Selwyn, R. G. (2014). FDG-PET imaging in mild traumatic brain injury: A critical review. *Frontiers in Neuroenergetics*, January 9; 5(13). https://doi.org/10.3389/fnene.2013.00013

Cho, S., Aminian, K., Li, C., Lang, A. E., Houle, S., & Strafella, A. P. (2017). Fatigue in Parkinson's disease: The contribution of cerebral metabolic changes. *Human Brain Mapping*, 38, 283–292.

Clark, A. L., Delano-Wood, L., Sorg, S. F., Werhane, M. L., Hanson, K. L., & Schiehser, D. M. (2017). Cognitive fatigue is associated with reduced anterior internal capsule integrity in veterans with history of mild to moderate traumatic brain injury. *Brain Imaging and Behavior*, 11(5), 1548–1554.

Cromwell, H. C., Mears, R. P., Wan, L., & Boutros, N. N. (2008). Sensory gating: A translational effort from basic to clinical science. *Clinical EEG and Neuroscience*, 39(2), 69–72.

Dello Russo, C., Boullerne, A. I., Gavrilyuk, V., Gavrilyuk, V., & Feinstein, D. L. (2004). Inhibition of microglial inflammatory responses by norepinephrine: Effects on nitric oxide and interleukin-1β production. *Journal of Neuroinflammation*, 9. https://doi.org/10.1186/1742-2094-1-9

DeLuca, J., Genova, H. M., Hillary, F. G., & Wylie, G. (2008). Neural correltates of cognitive fatigue in multiple sclerosis using fuctional MRI. *Journal of the Neurological Sciences*, 270, 28–39.

Dienel, G. A., & Cruz, N. F. (2016). Aerobic glycolysis during brain activation: Adrenergic regulation and influence of norepinephrine on astrocytic metabolism. *Journal of Neurochemistry*, 138, 14–52. https://doi.org/10.1111/jnc.13630

Dobryakova, E., Genova, H. M., DeLuca, J., & Wylie, G. R. (2015). The dopamine imbalance hypothesis of fatigue in multiple sclerosis and other neurological disorders. *Frontiers in Neurology*, 12(6), 52. https://doi.org/10.3389/fneur.2015.00052

Engström Nordin, L., Möller, M. C., Julin, P., Bartfai, A., Hashim, F., & Li, T.-Q. (2016). Post mTBI fatigue is associated with abnormal brain functional connectivity. *Scientific Reports*, 6(21183). https://doi.org/10.1038/srep21183

Erickson, M. A., Dohi, K., & Banks, W. A. (2012). Neuroinflammation: A common pathway in CNS diseases as mediated at the blood-brain barrier. *Neuroimmunomodulation*, 19(2), 121–130. https://doi.org/10.1159/000330247

Genova, H. M., Hillary, F. G., Wyliem, G., Rypma, B., & DeLuca, J. (2009). Examination of processing speed deficits in multiple sclerosis using functional magnetic resonance imaging. *Journal of the International Neuropsychological Society*, 15, 383–393.

Glavå, G., Skau, S., Lövdén, M., & Johansson, B. (2025). Differences in frontal cortical brain function between individuals suffering from pathological mental fatigue following acquired brain injury and healthy individuals. *Behavioural Brain Research*, 490(115631). https://doi.org/10.1016/j.bbr.2025.115631

Hammett, S. T., Cook, E., Hassan, O., Hughes, C.-A., Rooslien, H., Tizkar, R., & Larsson, J. (2020). GABA, noise and gain in human visual cortex. *Neuroscience Letters*, 736(135294). https://doi.org/10.1016/j.neulet.2020.135294

Hansson, E., & Rönnbäck, L. (2004). Altered neuronal-glial signaling in glutamatergic transmission as a unifying mechanism in chronic pain and mental fatigue. *Neurochemical Research*, 29, 989–996.

Harris, J. J., Jolivet, R., & Attwell, D. (2012). Synaptic energy use and supply. *Neuron Review*, 6(75,7), 762–777.

Johansson, B., & Rönnbäck, L. (2025). The Brain Fatigue Syndrome—Symptoms, probable definition, and pathophysiological mechanisms. *Journal of Clinical Medicine*, 14(3271). https://doi.org/10.3390/jcm14103271

Kohl, A. D., Wylie, G. R., Genova, H. M., Hillary, F., & DeLuca, J. (2009). The neural correlates of cognitive fatigue in traumatic brain injury using functional MRI. *Brain Injury*, 23(5), 420–432.

Magistretti, P. J., & Allaman, I. (2015). A cellular perspective on brain energy metabolism and fuctional imaging. *Neuron Review*, 86, 883–901.

McGuire, J. L., Ngwenya, L. B., & McCullumsmith, R. E. (2019). Neurotransmitter changes after traumatic brain injury: An update for new treatment strategies. *Molecular Psychiatry*, 24, 995–1012.

Mergenthaler, P., Lindauer, U., Dienel, G. A., & Meisel, A. (2013). Sugar for the brain: The role of glucose in physiological and pathological brain function. *Trends in Neurosciences*, 36(10), 587–597.

Raichle, M. E. (2015). The restless brain: How intrinsic activity organizes brain function. *Philosophical Transactions of the Royal Society*, 19;370(1668), 20140172. https://doi.org/10.1098/rstb.2014.0172

Ramage, A. E., Tate, D. F., New, A. B., Lewis, J. D., & Robin, D. A. (2019). Effort and fatigue-Related functional connectivity in mild traumatic brain injury. *Frontiers in Neurology*, 9, 1165. https://doi.org/10.3389/fneur.2018.01165

Rodrigues, R. J., Tomé, A. R., & Cunha, R. A. (2015). ATP as a multi-target danger signal in the brain. *Frontiers in Neurology*, 28 April. https://doi.org/10.3389/fnins.2015.00148

Roelcke, U., Kappos, L., Lechner-Scott, J., Brunnschweiler, H., Huber, S.W., Ammann, W., . . . Leenders, K. L. (1997). Reduced glucose metabolism in the frontal cortex and basal ganglia of multiple sclerosis patients with fatigue: A 18F-fluorodeoxyglucose positron emission tomography study *Neurology*, 48(6), 1566–1571.

Rönnbäck, L., & Hansson, E. (2004). On the potential role of glutamate transport in mental fatigue. *Journal of Neuroinflammation*, 1, 22.

Rönnbäck, L., & Johansson, B. (2022). Long-lasting pathological mental fatigue after brain injury–A dysfunction in glutamate neurotransmission? *Frontiers in Behavioral Neuroscience*, 15, 791984. https://doi.org/10.3389/fnbeh.2021.791984

Siracusa, R., Fusco, R., & Cuzzocrea, S. L. (2019). Astrocytes: Role and functions in brain pathologies. *Frontiers Pharmacology*, 10(1114). https://doi.org/10.3389/fphar.2019.01114

Skau, S., Bunketorp-Käll, L., Kuhn, H. G., & Johansson, B. (2019). Mental fatigue and functional near-infrared spectroscopy (fNIRS) – Based assessment of cognitive performance after mild traumatic brain injury. *Frontiers Human Neuroscience*, 13(145). https://doi.org/10.3389/fnhum.2019.00145

Skau, S., Jonsdottir, I. H., Sjörs Dahlman, A., Johansson, B., & Kuhn, H. G. (2021). Exhaustion disorder and altered brain activity in frontal cortex detected with fNIRS. *Stress and Health*, 24(1), 64–75.

Sundström, A., Marklund, P., Nilsson, L.-G., Cruts, M., Adolfsson, R., van Broeckhoven, C., & Nyberg, L. (2004). APOE influences on neuropsychological function after mild head injury within-person comparisons. *Neurology*, 62, 1963–1966.

Syková, E. (2004a). Diffusion properties of the brain in health and disease. *Neurochemistry*, 45, 453–466.

Syková, E. (2004b). Extrasynaptic volume transmission and diffusion parameters of extracellular space. *Neuroscience*, 129, 861–876.

Vergara, R. C., Jaramillo-Riveri, S., Luarte, A., Moënne-Loccoz, C., Fuentes, R., Couve, A., & Maldonado, P. E. (2019). The energy homeostasis principle: Neuronal energy regulation drives local network dynamics generating behavior. *Frontiers in Computational Neuroscience*, 13, 49. https://doi.org/10.3389/fncom.2019.00049

Wylie, G. R., E. Dobryakova, DeLuca, J., Chiaravalloti, N., Essad, K., & Genova, H. (2017). Cognitive fatigue in individuals with traumatic brain injury is associated with caudate activation. *Scientific Reports*, 7(8973). https://doi.org/10.1038/s41598-017-08846-6

Xia, Q.-P., Cheng, Z.-Y., & He, L. (2019). The modulatory role of dopamine receptors in brain neuroinflammation. *International Immunopharmacology*, November;76, 105908. https://doi.org/10.1016/j.intimp.2019.105908

Yudkoff, M., Nissim, I., Daikhin, Y., Lin, Z. P., Nelson, D., Pleasure, D., & Erecinska, M. (1993). Brain glutamate metabolism: Neuronal-astroglial relationships. *Developmental Neuroscience*, 15, 343–350.

Zielinski, M. R., Systrom, D. M., & Rose, N. R. (2019). Fatigue, sleep, and autoimmune and related disorders. *Frontiers in Immunology*, 10, 1827. https://doi.org/10.3389/fimmu.2019.01827

7 Treatment and support

No recommended treatment for Brain Fatigue syndrome exists today, and treatment options and studies are few. Despite this, patients report long-lasting brain fatigue as one of the most troublesome symptoms following an illness affecting the brain, having a huge impact on everyday activities, reducing quality of life, and diminishing the ability to work. One reason for this could be the ignorance of healthcare providers, who often assume brain fatigue to be an additional, non-priority factor. In contrast, the affected people want rehabilitation for fatigue to be prioritized.

Diagnosis-specific concerns should, of course, be treated so that functions such as physical, cognitive, linguistic, etc., can improve. In addition, everyday stimulation through various activities and social contacts is needed for well-being. However, everything must be adapted to the individual's energy budget to achieve a good outcome.

There is no approved drug to treat brain fatigue, but a few pharmacological studies have reported reduced fatigue or improved wakefulness, making the fatigue easier to manage. Additionally, a few non-pharmacological studies have reported reduced fatigue.

Even though we don't have an efficient cure for brain fatigue, we can't ignore it. Treatment options that can alleviate brain fatigue exist and can be used today. In this chapter, we will provide examples from our own experience and research, as well as other treatment alternatives.

We hope this chapter will contribute to increasing knowledge on how improvements can be achieved for those who suffer from brain fatigue and provide healthcare staff and others with alternatives for support and rehabilitation. It is important to start in the early phase, as there is a risk that patients may develop emotional and social problems later, which need to be avoided or managed as well as possible. Additionally, rehabilitation for brain fatigue needs to be accessible for a long time, as brain fatigue can be a long-lasting or chronic problem for many.

DOI: 10.4324/9781003732105-7

Knowledge and education

First, from both the personal perspective and that of healthcare providers, basic knowledge must be achieved. The reduced energy and ability to participate in daily activities must be understood, as well as the associated symptoms, and this must be done in a deeper sense. The personal stories embedded in this book can help with that. Lastly, it is important to listen to patients with care, curiosity, and an open mind.

Initially, after an injury or illness, there is hope that brain fatigue will quickly pass. This is also the case for many. For example, after a concussion or mild stroke, brain fatigue may disappear after a few weeks or months, but not for all. For others, it becomes more evident after being discharged from the hospital when trying to return to life before the illness. It is thus important to consistently screen for brain fatigue and provide proper education to patients and their carers. For those with long-lasting problems, it can be tough and a long process to find acceptance and meet life as it is. Support and care may be needed for many years. Additionally, relatives and friends also need to understand and learn. Furthermore, brain fatigue needs to be understood by the person suffering from it, as described below by a person after a concussion.

Personal story: The Brain Fatigue Syndrome needs to be understood

> I would describe brain fatigue as a kind of "invisible" illness, primarily because it doesn't show on "normally healthy" people that they have brain fatigue and suffer from it in their daily lives. Of course, brain fatigue exists in all its various stages among all different types of people with different types of problems, and it is certainly very sad to live with multiple illnesses. But what I (who many classify as a normal young healthy man without physical dysfunctions) have noticed is that a kind of strange barrier is created between the "healthy" person with brain fatigue and their surroundings. I remember this barrier as extremely stressful, and it made me feel even worse and confused about who I was. Suddenly, I had difficulty meeting friends/family in the same way as before, as they didn't understand why I felt the way I did. I often heard, "You look healthy... are you really sick?" They didn't understand what brain fatigue meant and that it can't be seen from the outside. I had difficulty explaining what my brain fatigue entailed, as it was new to me too and I had no knowledge of the illness. I felt what I felt in my body, but I couldn't explain why it was happening. I also couldn't describe when my difficulties might arise or why they suddenly appeared, and this created a kind of distrust among them (friends/family/healthcare) towards me and whether I was really telling the truth. For example, they

didn't believe that I suddenly needed to turn off the light, ask people to speak more quietly, that I couldn't meet for as long, that I constantly forgot things, that I couldn't work, or that I could suddenly respond in a strange way. And I didn't understand it either, but I knew I couldn't live as I had before. If I tried to live as I did before, I would suffer greatly later, with, for example, extreme headaches that lasted for many days and sometimes weeks. During many periods, I couldn't get out of bed because I didn't listen to what my body needed. An adjustment was needed, but I didn't know myself what should be done.

But everything changed when I met a neuropsychologist knowledgeable about what brain fatigue entails and has an ability to understand how illness can affect a person. The psychologist shared this knowledge with me, which changed my view of myself and my brain fatigue.

Brain fatigue exists among so many around us, yet knowledge about the illness is limited within healthcare. This limitation causes people with brain fatigue to suffer even more and end up in even greater pain. Understanding illness and informing healthcare about its impact is important, not only for the patient but for the whole society.

Long-term perspective

When suffering from brain fatigue, managing work and everyday life can be challenging. Often, the person has a strong will to regain their previous life. The desire exists, and they try to resume activities, but it doesn't work as it used to. It's not about a lack of interest, laziness, or apathy.

Doctors may find it difficult to understand the discrepancy between the patient's will and what is endurable over days and weeks, especially when the patient is unclear about their limits. This increases the risk of activity levels rising too quickly, which is particularly problematic when resuming work or increasing working hours. If the person pushes themselves too hard, it can lead to mental health problems and setbacks. When unable to handle all the impressions and demands, there is an increased risk of total mental exhaustion. Simultaneously, worry and despair may intensify, and some may become depressed and suffer from anxiety.

Go slow

Experience shows that activity levels must be increased very carefully, both at work and in everyday life. The pace of increasing activities must be adapted, possibly over several years. People have reported that after a few years, or maybe five, it gets better. This is promising, but it is not true for all. We can't provide prognostics on who will take either path based on current knowledge. Regardless of the scenario, brain fatigue needs to be managed. Life can improve. From the examples below, it is workable and possible. Support may be necessary for many, and for many years.

The personal ability to manage stress and frustration accompanying brain fatigue varies. Some have an inherent terrific coping ability, while others are totally lost and need a lot of support. In Western healthcare society, the overarching goal is to be more efficient and produce rehabilitation faster. However, with brain fatigue, improvement takes time, and no quick fix exists today.

Energy conservation strategies

Strategies to conserve mental energy are always necessary, regardless of the treatment methods used, as exemplified below. It is important to note that the strategies provided are just examples and can be helpful or serve as inspiration for other situations and circumstances. All strategies need to be adapted and individualized.

Using strategies to save energy in activities can help individuals participate in activities, but in an adapted way. The activity level must be balanced between rest and regaining energy, using mental energy sustainably. This should be in accordance with the personal energy budget. While this may sound simple, support may be necessary to figure out a balanced lifestyle. It is also challenging to be honest with oneself and truly understand what balanced living means, such as taking regular breaks during an activity and avoiding excessive disturbances like sound, noise, and stress. However, joyful and enjoyable activities must be included, even if they consume energy, as long as they can be balanced with restful activities.

It is not effective to use mental training activities, start working, or increase working hours to reduce brain fatigue. On the contrary, it may worsen the condition. Using working memory programmes may improve working memory in specific situations, but the transfer effect to daily life and functioning is questionable. Regardless, whatever we do in daily life is a practice of cognitive functions. The important thing is to use energy wisely.

The need for brain rest

We are constantly exposed to visual and auditory impressions in modern society, and the brain works continuously, needing help to calm down from time to time. Good brain rest is always important. Long-term experience has taught us that it is not possible to push too hard and increase activity too quickly. Increasing mental activity with the hope of improvement does not work if there isn't enough mental energy. Doing so poses a significant risk of worsening brain fatigue and resulting in mental exhaustion. Let it take time. Energy must endure over days, weeks, months, and years. Therefore, we advocate caution in returning to work and everyday routines. This does not imply avoiding activities. Sometimes, it is important for well-being to participate in social activities, even if they are demanding, as long as they are adapted to the energy budget. However, it can be difficult to know when to stop and rest. It is natural to be active when feeling more energetic and better. Activities also tend to be more manageable at that moment. Additionally, it is nearly impossible to feel the increase in brain fatigue during the activity and stop in time. There is often a delay before the person experiences the increase in brain fatigue, and sometimes it can appear very suddenly.

Sometimes, longer periods of calm and brain rest are needed during the day. Let activity periods also be interrupted with shorter breaks. The duration and frequency of these breaks are personal and may differ between activities. Pacing, or finding a personal balance between conserving energy/rest and the activity performed, has been shown to be beneficial for alleviating fatigue. It may be necessary to use an alarm initially, especially when engaging in fun and inspiring activities. Figure 7.1 illustrates this.

The better one understands their personal brain fatigue and can use brain rest and strategies, the more effective it can be. If the activity level is too high over a longer period, or if a situation induces more stress and exhaustion, brain fatigue can worsen. Figure 7.2 illustrates how brain fatigue can develop over time when pushing too hard and how it can improve when activities and daily living are better adapted. Be patient, it all takes time.

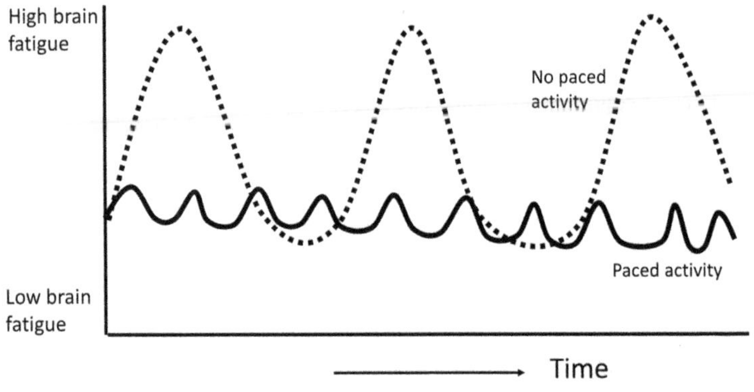

Figure 7.1 Pacing the activity can be helpful. With a non-paced activity pattern, the ups and downs will be significant, potentially leading to frustrating setbacks. In contrast, pacing the activity can create a more balanced and smoother activity rhythm with less frustration.

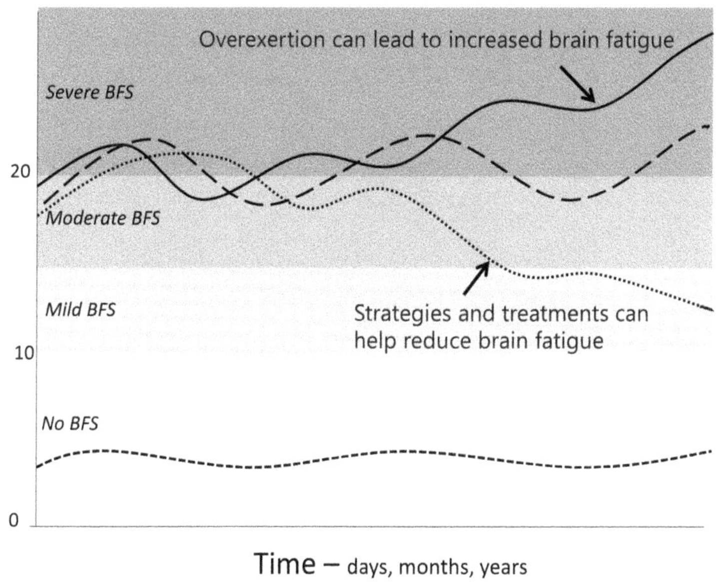

Figure 7.2 Adapting and using strategies for daily living and activities is helpful.

How to rest the brain

Walking in the forest or other natural environments or engaging in activities in nature when it is calm is reported by many who suffer from brain fatigue as nourishing and providing good brain rest (Figure 7.3). Maybe just sitting under a tree in a calm place, sitting by the lake, or watching birds. However, strong winds can be disturbing and energy-consuming. Handicrafts can also be helpful, as long as they are calm and don't require much attention, such as carving, embroidery, gardening, or painting. Meditation, yoga, tai chi, and qi gong can be beneficial. Sleep is always good for brain rest. Take these examples of brain rest as just examples. What is experienced as calming and helpful is personal. A walk in the forest can be overwhelming if there is too much to attend to. It all depends on the person and the situation. Everyone suffering from brain fatigue needs to find their own way to rest and save energy.

It is beneficial to personally experience the difference between a calm brain and an overloaded brain filled with impressions. Try this experiment: Can you feel the difference between sitting in a calm place, just watching a tree or nature in front of you, and then returning to a mental activity, perhaps surfing on your smartphone or listening to people? What is the difference? How does it feel in your brain and body?

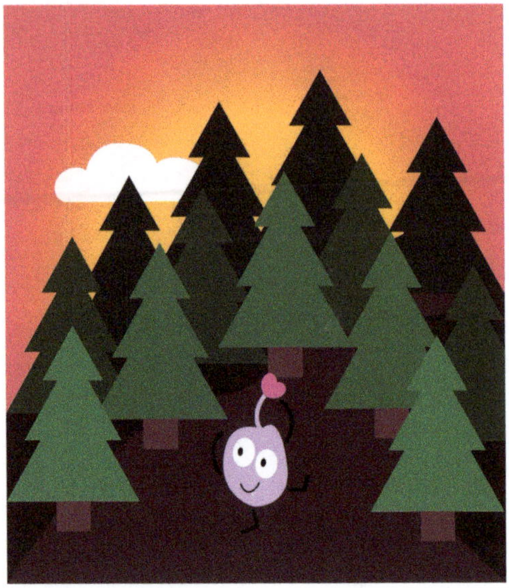

Figure 7.3 A moment in nature can bring calm and good brain rest.

Do the activity slower

How to adapt is personal. Taking several pauses while being active is helpful. It also matters how the activity is performed. Can the activity be done more calmly and relaxedly? Instead of rushing through, do the activity at a slower pace. For example, adapt the speed to a slower pace while eating, brushing teeth, reading, walking, cooking while stirring the pot, kneading dough, and other activities. This way of doing activities can be practised, focusing on one activity with awareness and not multitasking. Do not try to be efficient. Let it take time, and you may find that some activities can be done with pleasure and joy, and maybe with less energy.

Planning

Saving energy requires planning. Planning provides an overview and foresight and creates calm. It becomes clear if there are too many activities during the day and week. Brain rest also needs to be planned to ensure enough time for it during the day. An occupational therapist can help people get an overview of activities during the day and week and give advice on how to structure the days and weeks (Figure 7.4).

Alleviate sensitivity to sound and light

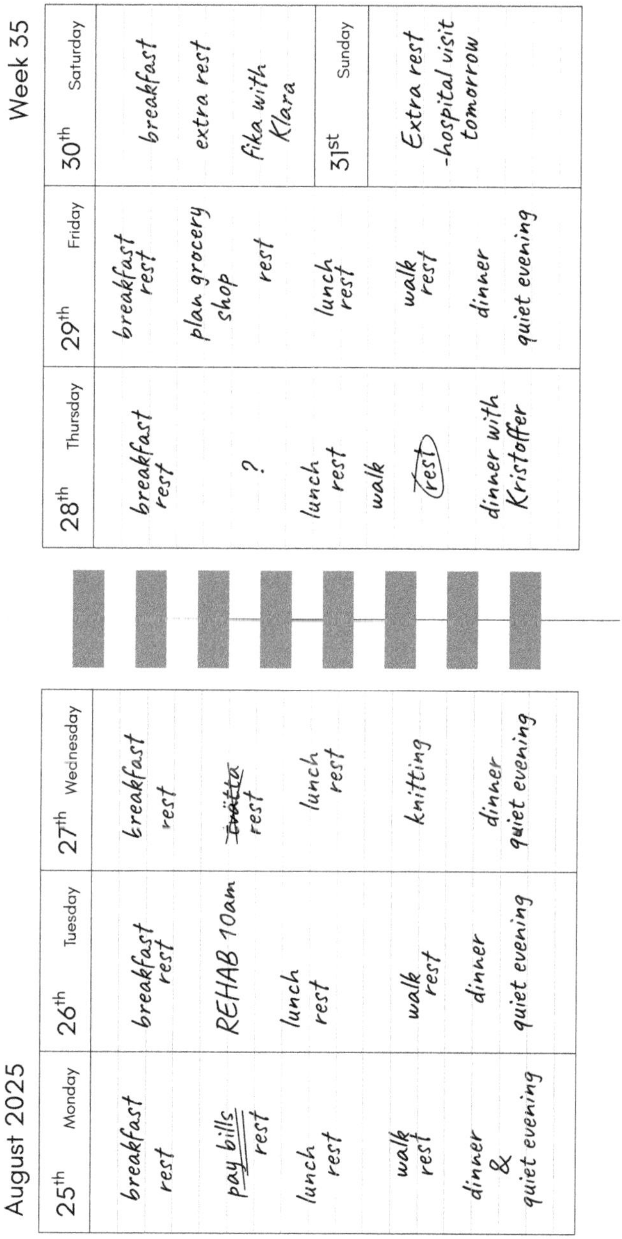

Figure 7.4 A calendar can be a helpful tool for planning your days and weeks.

Impressions from sound and light can be difficult to manage. Sound and light may be experienced as stronger than usual. Even smell can be a problem. As a help, the use of earplugs, sunglasses, or glasses filtering out blue and green wavelengths may be helpful for some, but not for all. The use of protection can be useful in situations when needed. Not all the time, but when going by bus or being in hectic and noisy environments, it can help save energy and use the energy on what is important.

Meetings and parties

Meetings and parties can be demanding, filled with many people and a lot of impressions. Still, it may be important to participate in a meeting. Suggest a time of day when your energy is higher. For many, it is difficult to follow the conversation and remember what was discussed or decided. Ask a friend or relative to join the meeting, take notes, and have someone to discuss the meeting with afterward. It can also be necessary to ask for a break during the meeting and to decide beforehand how long the meeting will last. If an appointment is planned, ask to have it written down on paper, sent via SMS, or emailed. This makes it possible to go back and check the time and date.

Attending a party, dinner, or just meeting friends is important for social belonging and stimulation. The sad thing is that it is extremely energy-demanding. One way to handle this is to prepare beforehand with extra rest and reserve time the day after for rest. It may be necessary to take a break during dinner or leave earlier. Planning in advance how long you can stay can be helpful. Inform others in advance about your plans. It is not about disliking the party, just a lack of energy. It will also be necessary to decline meetings if there are too many too close together or if they are expected to take too much energy. It is a personal balance between what is important and what is not. It is always important to find joy in life, even if low energy sets limits.

Shopping

Shopping is a common problem for those with brain fatigue. The bigger the shop, the worse it can be. Shops are filled with a lot of impressions, such as sounds, visual information, smells, and people moving around. However, it is necessary to buy food and other things, but it needs to be handled wisely. When visiting a shop, go at a time of day when there are fewer people around and decide beforehand to visit just one shop. If possible, choose a calm shop. Today, a lot can be bought online. It can be more calming to shop from home, taking time to choose without hurry. For some, using a computer can be too demanding, as it is also filled with impressions and information. Getting help from others may be necessary.

Travelling

Travelling short or long distances can be hard to manage. Buses, trains, and flights mean many people moving around with a lot of sounds and visual impressions. Even travelling by car can be overwhelming. Making the journey as calm as possible is necessary. Travelling by car without the radio on or asking others to talk less or not at all for a period can help. Using earplugs and covering the eyes can also be helpful. Travelling to a calm place, away from the demands of home, can provide insight and inspiration for managing brain fatigue better upon return.

Reading and writing

Reading is often regarded as relaxing, but for those suffering from brain fatigue, it is not an easy task. Many stop reading, read short parts, and become very tired easily. It can also be hard to understand and remember the content of the text when automatic functions are not working efficiently. Writing and spelling can also be more difficult. Spelling mistakes or writing down the wrong digits for time and date can lead to missed appointments. Healthcare providers should be curious and ask patients if reading a book or text works as before the illness. Ask how many pages they can read.

Audiobooks can work instead of reading, but not for everyone. Reading short parts, reading slowly, and not forcing the reading can be helpful, along with taking regular breaks. Start with easy books or even familiar ones. Read for fun, even if it is hard to remember the content later.

Sleep

Disturbed sleep is common among people suffering from brain fatigue. So far, there are no well-controlled studies indicating that sleep dysfunction explains brain fatigue. Undoubtedly, sleep is important, but problematic when suffering from brain fatigue. Sleep can be too short, interrupted, shallow, or too long, and in the morning, one may not feel refreshed. Better sleep quality often improves brain fatigue, but does not cure it.

It is important to have a regular day-night cycle, meaning waking up and going to bed at regular times. Finding a regular routine with activities and outdoor walks or other activities during the day can also be helpful. A nap during the day may be necessary, but it should be adapted to avoid interfering with night-time sleep. In the evening, try to calm down well in advance before going to bed. Calm the brain.

Sometimes medication is necessary, at least for a while. In general, consultation with a doctor to explore what medicine can give the best result is necessary. Even a combination of drugs, preferably in low doses, can be beneficial.

An interesting substance is melatonin. Melatonin is a hormone that regulates the circadian rhythm. Normally, darkness starts the production of melatonin in the pineal gland in the brain and induces sleep, while light causes that production to stop. However, in our clinical work, we have not found evidence to suggest melatonin for sleep problems after brain injury.

The general recommendation is to use caution with drugs containing benzodiazepines for people after brain injury due to their negative impact on cognition and possibly the healing process in the brain. It is also important to be careful and start with a low dose, as it is common to be more sensitive to psychotropic medications.

Pharmacological studies

Methylphenidate

Research to alleviate brain fatigue has been conducted to a very limited extent. However, we can state today that brain fatigue can be alleviated but not cured with the drugs explored so far. The addition of dopamine has shown the best effect in the few studies carried out. The effects of methylphenidate (Ritalin) and OSU6162 have been evaluated in people who have suffered a mild head injury or stroke and are well recovered, except for experiencing significant brain fatigue.

Our pharmacological studies are based on the theory described in this book. According to our hypothesis, an imbalance occurs in systems important for attention and concentration. Dopamine is a neurotransmitter or signalling substance that is crucial for attention. From animal studies, dopamine signalling is reduced in the brain when there is neuroinflammation affecting the neuronal network. Stimulating dopamine signalling and thereby activating ion pumps and transport systems for substances like glutamate may alleviate brain fatigue. The signalling substance norepinephrine, which has also been shown to decrease during neuroinflammation, is also of interest. Norepinephrine has been shown to increase both glutamate and glucose uptake, potentially improving nerve cell signalling efficiency along neural pathways in the brain and enhancing attention.

With methylphenidate, we found reduced mental fatigue in two-thirds of study participants. They reported less brain fatigue according to their ratings on the Mental Fatigue Scale, were able to start or initiate activities more easily, and performed better on neuropsychological tests measuring information processing and attention (Figure 7.5).

Participants who experienced good effects were allowed to continue with methylphenidate and were closely monitored over six years. We have shown long-term treatment effects with methylphenidate, but these effects appear to be reversible. The positive effect on brain fatigue is only seen

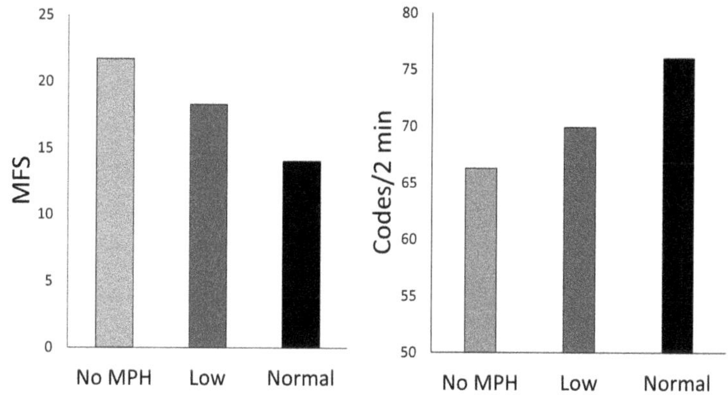

Figure 7.5 The left figure illustrates the reduction in brain fatigue (MFS rating) with no medication, a low dose, and a normal dose of methylphenidate (MPH). The right figure shows the improvement in processing speed (coding, WAIS), peaking at the normal dose.

during ongoing treatment with methylphenidate. When participants took a four-week break, their brain fatigue returned to a similar level as when they started with methylphenidate. This indicates that methylphenidate does not mediate healing or recovery of brain fatigue but can improve quality of life.

Our treatment proposals for methylphenidate are based on extensive research and experience with traumatic brain injury. While we cannot comment on its effectiveness for brain fatigue from other conditions, it's important to note that methylphenidate may not always be the best option. Other medications might be relevant too.

Years of experience and knowledge have taught us that competent and responsible drug treatment requires solid expertise and close patient contact. When brain fatigue becomes prolonged or chronic, treatment with methylphenidate should enhance quality of life without causing side effects. Therefore, individual dose adjustments and careful patient follow-up are crucial.

We recommend considering methylphenidate if brain fatigue persists for over a year. However, starting treatment too early can be counterproductive, as the brain's natural recovery period can be lengthy. Patients must first understand their brain fatigue and learn energy-conserving strategies, which remain necessary even with medication.

A medical assessment is essential to determine if medication is a viable treatment option for brain fatigue, considering that some conditions may not be suitable for such treatment.

Before starting treatment

- Tests and Sampling: Blood pressure, heart rate, ECG, and blood tests.
- Subjective Tests: Self-assessment forms for brain fatigue (MFS), depression, and anxiety.
- Objective Tests: Neuropsychological tests focusing on speed and attention.

Starting treatment

Begin with a low dose, gradually increasing over two to three weeks. Individual responses vary, and both short- and long-acting methylphenidate are available. In our study, short-acting methylphenidate was initially used to set the individual dose more easily. Most people find a dose of 60 mg/day (divided into three doses of 20 mg each) effective, but adjustments may be necessary. Close patient contact is vital, with telephone check-ins and return visits within a month recommended. Inform patients about common side effects and adjust the dose if needed.

Follow-up visits

- Discuss effects and side effects.
- Measure blood pressure and heart rate.
- Have patients complete self-assessments for brain fatigue (MFS), depression, and anxiety.
- Conduct neuropsychological tests for processing speed and attention.
- Schedule regular follow-up visits, more frequently at the beginning, and ensure patients can call if needed.
- Take a four-week break annually to evaluate the continued need for medication.

Long-term treatment experience

Life changes, such as increased stress, can affect the efficacy of methylphenidate. Some patients may not experience benefits during stressful periods but might find it helpful later. Reviewing the patient's life situation and providing support and rehabilitation before testing methylphenidate can be valuable. Our experience shows that while methylphenidate can reduce brain fatigue, it requires balancing activity and rest. The energy deficiency is not cured.

Our long-term experience indicates that the initial dose usually remains effective without the need for higher doses.

Positive effects

Research shows that methylphenidate can reduce brain fatigue, depression, and anxiety symptoms and improve cognition. Many patients report improved sleep, better pain management, and cognitive improvements, such as clearer thinking and better concentration. They also report reduced stress sensitivity and find it easier to initiate activities. As one patient said, "I've got my life back." However, patients must continue to manage their mental energy limits.

Side effects

Side effects are typically dose-dependent and transient, such as dry mouth and palpitations, which can be managed by adjusting the dose. Common reasons for discontinuing treatment include restlessness, anxiety, palpitations, increased blood pressure, and depressive symptoms. Some patients may not feel any effect and choose not to continue. Long-term follow-ups show no additional side effects, with heart rate and blood pressure remaining within normal ranges and no ECG changes. Weight changes were minimal. Methylphenidate works well for some but not for others.

When effective, methylphenidate can alleviate brain fatigue and improve overall quality of life. Here is a personal story.

The incident

I slipped on an ice patch and hit the back of my head hard on December 28, 2009. I don't remember the fall itself but recall a terrifying roar in my head when I was lying on the ground. It subsided after a while. For two weeks, I had to stay still. I had a constant headache. I was dizzy. I developed tinnitus after the blow, which sounds like TV static or crickets. I had great difficulty sleeping at first, even sleeping pills didn't work. I became very sensitive to noise. I repeatedly made spelling mistakes on the computer. I completely lost my ability to think when I started to get tired.

The progression

I started working after a while, first at 25 percent and then increasing, and was pressured by the Social Insurance Agency to start full-time after the vacation, around July 1, 2010. I was working uphill, so to speak. After a while, it became harder and harder to function full-time. I went to the health center and reduced my working hours, first to 75 percent, then to 50 percent. Due to noise sensitivity, I had to get earplugs for noisy environments, such as large stores, lunch restaurants, music services, concerts, and family dinners.

I was at a rehabilitation centre. It was a wonderful experience to meet people who knew what it was about. Later, I met research on brain injury and Ritalin (methylphenidate) through my wife, who is a general practitioner. I didn't join the research group itself but felt I was treated almost as if I were. I took tests and had regular meetings at the hospital. I received Ritalin, which significantly improved my quality of life. I could focus much better, both at work and in social life. The latest caseworker at the Social Insurance Agency treated me very well and with respect. She believed in me and my doctors. She asked the questions she needed based on the agency's rules but didn't pressure me and realized that it didn't matter what I did; worked, painted the house, did carpentry, socialized, sailed, or travelled. I still had to withdraw at least a couple of times a day to rest.

Eventually, I understood that I needed to retire two years earlier than planned due to my injury. I simply didn't function well enough. I worked 50 percent in the last period, but since I was a manager with staff responsibility, operational responsibility, and financial responsibility, it was difficult, even though I had an assistant manager by my side. Additionally, it is very difficult to get another 100 percent position if I am to be on sick leave 50 percent.

Living with brain fatigue

I was previously a very active person. Worked a lot and engaged in various activities. There was no chance at all to continue like that. I mostly have a good mood, which helps me a lot. I have a good home life and a good social life with family and friends. I also have good interests that add a lot to my life. Still, I had some depressing months one winter when I worked on realizing that I am now a disabled person. That I really had to redefine my self-image. It was a tough time. I still have dips, but not in the same way. I also heard from people who know me well, "Strange to see you so different now."

I am different compared to before. Life is different. The injury has affected my entire life and limited my life. My accident insurance company assessed this as minor, frighteningly incorrect assessment. Now I really must plan and balance my time. Plan and balance. Try to think in advance how the scenario might be – work/social life – rest – work/social life – rest. To this comes "How do I now explain to them that I can't manage? Who will I meet? How will they take it? How much should I say? Now I have to decline a trip, a meeting, a party again…" Think of how many people I can't meet as before, those I might have lunch or coffee with occasionally, and now haven't met for months or years. How can I plan that too? If I do one thing during the day, can I do another? Priorities make, for example, the grandchildren the most important – naturally! But I miss the lunches and coffee with these people. If I work or do something socially fun in the evening, it costs a longer rest period during the day and often an extra rest the following day when I am exhausted. Sometimes I consciously go beyond my limits and know that the next day I will be exhausted, but do it because I need it. My life needs it, and not least my grandchildren need it.

I often refrain from things I like and did before, like some concerts and parties. Sometimes I go for a while only with earplugs. Sometimes I go home earlier or make sure there is a room where I can rest, with earplugs. The earplugs are with me at lunch restaurants, etc. I have to avoid going into large stores. Sometimes I can almost feel panic in such environments. The earplugs are fantastic, but I can't keep up with conversations with several people at the table as I could before. I have to concentrate on one or two.

I participated in a rehabilitation group, the spring of 2018. There I got good tips, good thoughts, and help with structuring my days. One of the most important things was to put into words how I really feel. I would formulate the words for others, but it became equally important to formulate them for myself. A very strong experience and useful. It became clear to me that I no longer have any completely good days. Some can be better and others worse, but none are completely good. It was strong and emotional for me to realize and accept that. It was also something for some of my friends to understand who hadn't quite grasped the extent of what my injury means. That life is so different and limited for me now. It's tough that so many have such a hard time understanding or accepting what I say. They might want to comfort by saying, "I'm also more tired with age," and so on, but for me, it expresses that they don't take it in. And it happens all the time. And constantly trying to explain what isn't visible, over and over again. I don't always understand myself and my reactions either.

It's an uphill battle for us with brain fatigue that so few doctors are knowledgeable about how we feel. It's really bad that the Social Insurance Agency and their doctors don't realize how we feel. Sometimes I wonder about the ethics of these doctors. You are completely down but still have to fight. The energy isn't there. I know people who are much younger than I am, who aren't retirees, and who are completely broken by fights with the Social Insurance Agency.

There are no signs that the brain is getting better now after 9 years. I have to prepare for the future to be like this. I have to work on planning and balancing and hope that people, and I myself, can cope with me as I am today and even tomorrow.

Comment: In Sweden, Ritalin is officially prescribed only for ADHD. When the study concluded, all participants had to discontinue their Ritalin treatment.

Dopamine stabilizer OSU6162

In Parkinson's disease, certain brain areas lack dopamine, while in schizophrenia, dopamine levels in specific signalling systems are too high. Traditionally, treatments have aimed to increase dopamine in Parkinson's and decrease it in schizophrenia. However, to minimize the side effects of these drastic changes, researchers considered developing drugs that "stabilize" dopamine levels instead. Brain cells function best with stable signalling, neither too much nor too little dopamine is ideal.

Synthesized substances have shown a stabilizing effect on dopamine levels, though some critics argue that these effects are more about specific receptor systems than true stabilization. Aripiprazole, for example, inhibits one type of dopamine receptor while stimulating another, earning it the label of a partial dopamine receptor stimulator. It also affects serotonin receptors, stimulating one group while inhibiting another, thus acting as a stabilizer for both dopamine and serotonin systems.

OSU6162 and ACR16 are two other stabilizers with slightly different effects from aripiprazole. OSU6162, in particular, appears to stabilize both dopamine and serotonin systems. Since dopamine is crucial for attention and serotonin for emotions, studying these substances' effects on brain fatigue is highly relevant.

In two studies, a pilot and a follow-up, we investigated OSU6162's effect on brain fatigue. This drug is not yet on the market. Participants, who had long-term brain fatigue following brain injury or stroke, were otherwise well-rehabilitated. We found that OSU6162 had a milder effect on brain fatigue compared to methylphenidate. The studies, as well as others, reported mixed results: some participants experienced reduced fatigue and improved daily activity, while others saw no effect compared to placebo. Brain imaging (fMRI) showed that OSU6162 treatment normalized brain signalling compared to healthy controls.

Treatment with OSU6162, like methylphenidate, does not work for everyone. OSU6162 causes fewer side effects and is milder than methylphenidate. While methylphenidate may help some patients, it is not suitable for everyone, especially those with certain medical or psychiatric conditions. OSU6162, though less potent, may provide relief for some patients.

Additionally, based on our theory of the glutamate/GABA-glutamine cycle, GABA may deplete its transmitter pool, potentially contributing to the pathology of brain fatigue. This depletion could impair the brain's ability to suppress irrelevant information, which may help explain why individuals with brain fatigue often report difficulty filtering out redundant noise and feeling overwhelmed by sensory input.

Possible other medications

Studies have shown that modafinil can increase daytime alertness but it does little to improve concentration or brain fatigue. However, it has been effective in reducing excessive daytime sleepiness. For multiple sclerosis patients, amantadine reduced fatigue, but modafinil did not. Another study found that amantadine, modafinil, and methylphenidate were not superior to placebo in reducing fatigue in multiple sclerosis. amantadine, which increases dopamine signalling, has some effect on brain fatigue and may be worth trying.

Abilify, a dopamine stabilizer, has some similarities to OSU6162 but works differently. Both have milder effects compared to methylphenidate. When using Abilify for brain fatigue, very low doses are essential. Some patients benefit from combining methylphenidate with Abilify, experiencing both the powerful effect of methylphenidate and the gentle effect of low-dose Abilify. Combining methylphenidate with a dopamine agonist can also be beneficial, based on clinical experience.

Memantine, used for dementia, regulates glutamate signalling in the brain and reduces available glutamate in the synapse area. It may be worth trying at a low dose for brain fatigue, though its effect is limited. The combination of an opioid agonist and antagonist is intriguing based on cell culture studies, which show increased activity of certain ion pumps and enhanced glutamate use by astrocytes in neuroinflammation. Unfortunately, its effect on brain fatigue after head injury or stroke appears limited.

Acetylcholinesterase inhibitors did not reduce fatigue after TBI in a small study, while from an open-label study, participants reported increased vigilance.

Irritability and emotional instability

Clinical experience suggests that irritability and emotional instability, or tearfulness, can be treated with low-dose antidepressants like SSRIs if necessary. While fluoxetine did not reduce fatigue after stroke, it did improve depression symptoms. It's important to understand that irritability and tearfulness can worsen with increased brain fatigue, signalling the need for rest and reduced activities or working hours. As mental energy is regained, these symptoms will lessen. Relatives and close friends should be involved to help reduce or avoid unnecessary conflicts.

Through our treatment studies, we have gained significant insights into mental fatigue and received valuable information from participants. Unfortunately, there is still a lack of effective medical treatments for brain energy deficiency.

Treatment programmes

Mindfulness

Our research on mindfulness for brain fatigue has utilized the Mindfulness-Based Stress Reduction (MBSR) programme. This globally recognized programme, with its psychoeducative approach, has been extensively researched. We aim to share our insights on how mindfulness can alleviate fatigue, improve mental health, and help individuals better understand and accept life as it is. Mindfulness is not about rapid change but about learning to live life on its own terms, with acceptance and compassion. This approach contrasts with the high-pressure, quick-return-to-work demands of Western medical-driven healthcare.

The MBSR programme

Developed by Jon Kabat-Zinn in 1979, MBSR has been adapted for Western society as a complement to medical and mental health care. Over the years, the programme has been refined through personal experience, experimentation, and research. MBSR has been used for various patient groups and has clear guidelines for content and teacher education.

Kabat-Zinn defines mindfulness as "being aware through paying attention on purpose in a very special way: with intention, in the present moment, and without valuing or judging." It involves cultivating inner attitudes of presence, attention, compassion, caution, kindness, patience, and non-striving, all in the service of self-understanding and wisdom. Mindfulness helps us manage our lives more beneficially, providing opportunities to stop, calm down, and be aware of our current thoughts, feelings, and surroundings. It is about acting and making wise choices in the present moment, not in the past or future.

Mindfulness encompasses more than meditation; it is about living life insightfully and balanced, with self-care. The MBSR programme can help alleviate suffering and challenges after medical or psychological conditions, aiming to improve well-being. It is an educational programme that encourages meeting oneself wisely in the present moment. Mindfulness should never be demanding or stressful, and it should not have specific goals to achieve. The intention is to do something helpful without striving.

Learning to live in a new way can be necessary, and mindfulness can be an alternative treatment option for brain fatigue. However, mindfulness does not suit everyone. In cases of severe anxiety or acute illness, mindfulness may not be suitable. However, some may find relief using meditation at an early stage. For example, a participant in our first MBSR study found the body scan meditation helpful after suffering another concussion.

What is included in the MBSR programme

The MBSR programme provides a helpful start in mindfulness practice. It consists of eight weekly meetings, each lasting 2–2.5 hours, depending on the number of participants, and includes a full-day retreat between meetings six and seven. The programme incorporates meditations such as body scanning, sitting meditations, and gentle yoga. It also includes group reflections on practices and central themes for each meeting. Participants are encouraged to practise daily meditations and complete home assignments to better understand their lives and ways of living.

The MBSR programme is conducted in a face-to-face group setting, allowing participants to share experiences and support each other. This sharing is crucial, as it helps participants feel less alone and more understood. The themes and discussions during the programme are described as the "heart of the course," and the entire programme is imbued with compassion.

MBSR and Brain Fatigue Syndrome

Research has shown that MBSR can relieve stress, depression, anxiety, pain, and fatigue. It can also improve quality of life and serve as a treatment option for those suffering from prolonged discomfort after brain disorders. Mindfulness can enhance concentration, attention, and cognitive flexibility. Researchers have also observed changes in the brain, although the impact on behaviour is less clear.

Compassion is a central aspect of mindfulness. It involves kindness to oneself and others and understanding that it is universal. We often focus on life's hardships, but we all have the capacity for kindness and compassion, much like comforting a crying child. However, this skill may need practice.

Our findings

Our research group has found that mindfulness can alleviate brain fatigue and improve attention, as measured by cognitive tests. Meditation lasting about 45 minutes can be effective, providing time to calm down and be in silence. Initially, shorter meditations may be helpful, with the duration increasing over time. The body scan meditation can be challenging, as many participants fall asleep at first, but this improves later.

Participants were also able to manage the full-day retreat, a day of silence without communication, which allows for extended calmness.

It is difficult to pinpoint which part of the MBSR programme is most effective. Different participants benefit from different aspects. Many find the brain rest provided by meditation helpful, as well as the practice of slowing down daily activities. Understanding behavioural patterns and learning to act in ways that relieve stress and anxiety can also be beneficial. Some meditations focus on sounds, and several participants reported reduced sensitivity to noise after the course.

The emotional burden we add to suffering can be addressed through mindfulness. Sharing experiences and learning from each other is an essential part of the MBSR programme. This often-overlooked aspect of treatment programmes can help participants feel less lonely and recognize themselves in others. An interview study revealed that participants gained insight into their difficulties, became more compassionate, and found sharing experiences with others important. For most participants, it was a new way of relating to difficulties and coping with life more mindfully.

MBSR does not perform miracles, but it can improve life and help participants choose new paths and ways of dealing with challenges. The programme provides a "toolbox" that can be used in various ways, with different tools chosen at different times.

We have also found that it is possible to join an MBSR programme live online. In our study, the entire MBSR programme for people with brain fatigue was offered online, with participants meeting at the same time via the internet with a microphone and webcam. Internet programmes can be an option for those living far from a face-to-face group or unable to participate in a mindfulness programme for various reasons. For some, it may be safer to stay at home, while others may prefer meeting the group in person. We are all different!

Additionally, we evaluated the feasibility of a self-study MBSR online programme, as it can be challenging to participate in a face-to-face MBSR programme. People may live far from where a course is delivered, need to wait for a group to start, or have preferences for specific days and times. Some prefer to do the MBSR programme alone at home. However, they miss the discussion and sharing experiences with other group members, which is central to mindfulness. This may explain why half of the participants discontinued the course. They may have needed more support from a face-to-face group with weekly meetings. However, those who continued could follow the basic curriculum and reported reduced brain fatigue. The advantage of a self-study MBSR course is the flexibility to divide sessions, repeat parts, and adjust the time between sessions to personal needs.

After our first MBSR study, participants wanted more mindfulness, leading to the development of an in-depth programme called "Train4You." This programme is based on the Brahma Viharas, meditative practices known for cultivating four mental states: compassion, loving-kindness, appreciative joy, and equanimity. The group met once a month for eight sessions. We also offered the same advanced programme live online and compared it with a face-to-face group, finding improved self-compassion in both groups. Building a meditation routine takes time, and a longer practice period can provide inspiration, in-depth knowledge of mindfulness, and growth in acceptance.

Adapting MBSR to Brain Fatigue Syndrome

When teaching participants suffer from brain fatigue, certain challenges need to be addressed. They require a slower pace in everything, such as speaking more slowly, repeating messages, shorter talks, and more breathing space.

Starting a new activity like meditating can be daunting, especially if the meditation feels too long, such as a 45-minute body scan. Offer shorter meditations as alternative options, especially in the beginning, and encourage participants to gradually increase the duration.

Finding calm in meditation can be difficult when thoughts and impressions are distracting, which is even more problematic when brain fatigue is severe. Emphasize the principles of non-striving, non-judging, and simply doing. Perfection is not the goal.

We have not conducted studies comparing long and short meditations, but both are likely helpful for brain fatigue. People can use them according to what suits them best. Shorter meditations or breathing spaces during the day, even between activities, provide regular rest and time to reflect. However, longer meditation, as in the MBSR programme, can be beneficial. It takes time to calm down, and staying in that calmness can provide nourishing brain rest. The 45-minute meditation also allows people to dedicate time to their practice, saying, "This is for me."

The whole-day retreat offers the opportunity to explore what can happen during an extended period of calm. It is possible to attend, but participants need support. Discovering how to do activities at a slower pace with fewer impressions throughout the day can provide valuable insights. Some may feel calmer and more energized after a retreat, while others may become more fatigued.

Adapting the position for comfort is essential for both body and mind.

Encouragement and support are crucial. Meeting others in similar situations is helpful, even if discussions are tiring. Interrupt discussions with shorter meditations and keep the group small, no more than 10–15 participants.

It may be possible to find meditation groups locally or online. For those wanting to deepen their practice, a mindfulness course is beneficial. It's important to inquire about the mindfulness instructor's education and experience with brain fatigue. When dealing with brain fatigue and emotional problems, the teacher must have professional skills to meet these challenges and adapt the teaching accordingly.

Starting something new can be difficult when suffering from brain fatigue, as initiation is often reduced. Group meetings can be helpful initially. For those who want to further explore mindfulness and maintain their practice, an advanced programme over a longer period can provide great support and inspiration. This is especially important when dealing with mental illness, fatigue, or other health conditions, as building a regular mindfulness practice takes time. Meditation requires continuous practice, much like physical activity to maintain fitness.

A brain fatigue and mindfulness course (BF-M)

From our experience with the MBSR programme, we designed and evaluated a brain fatigue and mindfulness course. The Brain Fatigue and Mindfulness programme (BF-M) consists of six biweekly meetings, each lasting 2 hours, over 11 weeks. This schedule allows more time between meetings and extends the course duration. Each meeting includes meditation practice and knowledge about brain fatigue. The course begins with understanding brain fatigue and exploring how it affects the brain and body. It continues with practices for a deeper understanding of emotions and reactions, finding a balance between rest and activity. Group discussions and reflections on specific themes are included, allowing participants to share experiences and learn from each other (Table 7.1).

Participants receive pre-recorded meditations, including body scan, sitting meditation (20 and 45 minutes), breathing space, compassion meditation, and mountain meditation. They can also watch videos about brain fatigue and common symptoms after session one and strategies for managing brain fatigue after session four. The programme is conducted at a slower pace with repeated information. Shorter breaks with meditations are included as needed, and longer meditations during meetings provide

Table 7.1 Schematic presentation of the brain fatigue and mindfulness course

Session	*Meditations*	*Themes*
1	Body scan, 45 min	Central and common symptoms
2	Body scan, Breathing space	Explore brain fatigue
3	Sitting meditation 20 min, Breathing space	Explore emotions
4	Sitting meditation 45 min, Breathing space	Helpful strategies
5	Compassion meditation, Breathing space	What is helpful
6	Mountain meditation, Breathing space	The way forward

brain rest. The intention is to improve knowledge, increase insight into brain fatigue and emotional reactions, and learn to cope with difficulties in a friendlier way, meeting life on its own terms with compassion.

The BF-M course was evaluated with participants who had long-term brain fatigue from either an acquired brain injury or multiple sclerosis. We found reduced brain fatigue compared to controls after the course. Qualitative interviews revealed that the course provided an important opportunity to exchange and share experiences related to brain fatigue, feel understood, and feel less alone. Participants reported learning about their brain fatigue, reactions, and needs, gaining better acceptance of their problems. The programme also provided methods to manage and cope with brain fatigue in everyday life. They used meditations and adapted strategies to their needs. Overall, the programme shows promise, not as a miraculous cure, but as a way to provide new insights and strategies for better managing brain fatigue and its emotional burden. Hopefully, participants will be better prepared to manage their resources and limitations in the future. The programme needs to be explored with more participants and other patient groups, and it is important to find ways to attract more men, as currently about 75% of participants are women, similar to the MBSR programme worldwide.

Other treatment options

Mindfulness-based therapy for managing fatigue

A programme similar to BF-M for managing fatigue has been developed by Fiona McKechnie. This programme, based on Mindfulness-Based Cognitive Therapy, is adapted for fatigue and includes biweekly meetings, meditations, and group reflections. It has been used for participants with chronic fatigue.

Fatigue management course

The Fatigue Management Course is designed for patients suffering from general fatigue. Its goal is to help participants understand fatigue, how it affects daily life, and how to manage it with strategies tailored to their personal energy budget. This programme is commonly used for patients with multiple sclerosis and was initially developed for post-polio. It is a six-week course with weekly group meetings.

Step-by-step fatigue programme

Alex Howard emphasizes the importance of understanding fatigue and adapting methods to personal aspects of life. His step-by-step method takes several years but aims to improve sustainability according to existing energy levels. He addresses both physiological and psychological factors, primarily for chronic fatigue.

Cognitive behavioural therapy

Psychological treatments like Cognitive Behavioural Therapy (CBT) can positively impact and alleviate fatigue. CBT has been shown to improve sleep, daily fatigue levels, and depression symptoms. However, CBT cannot be standardized and must be adapted for individuals with brain fatigue.

Blue light therapy

Blue light therapy in the morning aims to effectively stop melatonin production and reduce sleepiness. Melatonin is a natural hormone that increases in the evening to induce sleep and decreases in the morning with light exposure. Researchers reported reduced daytime sleepiness and suggested that improving the circadian rhythm may alleviate fatigue. An in-home blue light study for reducing fatigue and daytime sleepiness after TBI showed no improvement in fatigue but did improve sleep patterns, reducing sleep disturbances and insomnia.

Neurophysiological therapeutic techniques

Neurophysiological treatments such as transcranial direct current stimulation (tDCS) and transcranial magnetic stimulation (TMS) have been investigated for their potential to alleviate fatigue, with varying results. tDCS, when compared to sham stimulation, has shown a reduction in post-stroke fatigue. However, combining tDCS with cognitive training did not yield additional beneficial effects for fatigue in stroke and multiple sclerosis (MS). TMS has been reported to be safe and effective in reducing fatigue in individuals with MS. In contrast, fatigue may interfere with the therapeutic effects of TMS on depression and anxiety in individuals with Long COVID. Despite methodological heterogeneity and differences in study design, neurophysiological techniques may hold promise for alleviating fatigue, as they aim to modulate brain activity and neural connectivity. Nevertheless, further research is needed to evaluate their efficacy in the treatment of Brain Fatigue Syndrome.

Physical activity

Physical activity is generally beneficial for health and well-being, but how it can be adapted for those suffering from fatigue is still unclear. For individuals with low physical activity before illness, introducing physical activity may alleviate fatigue. Whether fitness or strength training is more effective remains uncertain. Those who were physically active before illness often report that they cannot perform at the same level. Shorter walks, reduced running distances, or limited exercise time may be necessary to avoid increased brain fatigue. Graded activity training may be possible but needs to be adapted. A study combining graded activation with cognitive therapy showed a slight reduction in fatigue after stroke, but no significant difference between graded activation and cognitive therapy alone. Physical activity is important for well-being but must be tailored to each individual and their brain fatigue. Support from a physiotherapist can be beneficial.

Diet

Many people inquire about the importance of diet and dietary supplements, but there is no current evidence that any specific diet or supplement helps with brain fatigue. While many products are marketed to alleviate fatigue and cognitive impairment, pathological fatigue is challenging to improve, even with potent medication. We can only advocate for a healthy and balanced diet.

Treatment summary

Today, we can alleviate brain fatigue through education about brain fatigue, energy-saving strategies, sleep problem management, and emotional relief. This knowledge is crucial.

No drug currently cures long-term brain fatigue, but pharmacological treatments show promise for alleviating it. Non-pharmacological interventions can also alleviate brain fatigue. More research is needed to identify recommended drugs or treatment programmes.

Meeting others in similar situations can provide relief, as those suffering from brain fatigue often report loneliness and isolation due to their inability to join regular social activities. Feeling understood is also important. Non-governmental organizations for patient groups can offer support. Relatives and close friends need to be involved and supported, as we all live in connection with others.

Bibliography

Askari, S., Harvey, K., & Sam-Odutola, M. (2024). Patients experience of cognitive fatigue post-stroke: An exploratory study. *Disability and Rehabilitation*, 46(19), 4514–4521. https://doi.org/10.1080/09638288.2023.2280065

Barakou, I., Sakalidis, K. E., Abonie, U. S., Finch, T., Hackett, K. L., & Hettinga, F. J. (2023). Effectiveness of physical activity interventions on reducing perceived fatigue among adults with chronic conditions: A systematic review and meta-analysis of randomised controlled trials. *Scientific Reports*, 13(14582). https://doi.org/10.1038/s41598-023-41075-8

Berginström, N., Nordström, P., Ekman, U., Eriksson, J., Nyberg, L., & Nordström, A. (2019). Pharmaco-fMRI in patients with traumatic brain injury: A randomized controlled trial with the monoaminergic stabilizer (-)-OSU6162. *Journal of Head Trauma Rehabilitation*, 34(3), 189–198. https://doi.org/10.1097/HTR.0000000000000440

Berginström, N., Nordström, P., Schuit, R., & Nordström, A. (2017). The effects of (-)-OSU6162 on chronic fatigue in patients with traumatic brain injury: A randomized controlled trial. *Journal of Head Trauma Rehabilitation*, 32(2), E46–E54.

Carlsson, M. L., Burstein, E. S., Kloberg, A., Hansson, S., Schedwin, A., Nilsson, M., . . . Carlsson, A. (2011). I. In vivo evidence for partial agonist effects of (-)-OSU6162 and (+)-OSU6162 on 5-HT2A serotonin receptors. *Journal of Neural Transmission*, 118(11), 1511–1522.

Casson, S., Jones, M. D., Cassar, J., Kwai, N., Lloyd, A. R., Barry, B. K., & Sandler, C. X. (2023). The effectiveness of activity pacing interventions for people with chronic fatigue syndrome: A systematic review and meta-analysis. *Disability and Rehabilitation*, 45(23), 3788–3802. https://doi.org/10.1080/09638288.2022.2135776

Charvet, L., Goldberg, J. D., Li, X., Best, P., Lustberg, M., Shaw, M., . . . Krupp, L. (2025). Home-based transcranial direct current stimulation paired with cognitive training to reduce fatigue in multiple sclerosis. *Scientific Reports*, 15, 4551. https://doi.org/10.1038/s41598-025-88255-2

Choi-Kwon, S., Choi, J., Kwon, S. U., Kang, D.-W., & Kim, J. S. (2007). Fluoxetine is not effective in the treatment of post-stroke fatigue: A double-blind, placebo-controlled study. *Cerebrovascular Diseases*, 23(2–3), 103–108. https://doi.org/10.1159/000097045

Connolly, L. J., Rajaratnam, S. M. W., Murray, J. M., Spitz, G., Lockley, S. W., & Ponsford, J. L. (2021). Home-based light therapy for fatigue following acquired brain injury: A pilot randomized controlled trial. *BMC Neurology*, 21(1), 262. https://doi.org/10.1186/s12883-021-02292-8

Crane, R. S., Callen-Davies, R., Francis, A., Francis, D., Gibbs, P., Mulligan, B., . . . Vallejo, Z. (2023). Mindfulness-based stress reduction for our time: A curriculum that is up to the task. *Global Advances in Integrative Medicine and Health*, 12, 1–10. https://doi.org/10.1177/27536130231162604

Dong, X. L., Sun, X., Sun, W. M., Yuan, Q., Yu, G. H., Shuai, L., & Yuan, Y. F. (2021). A randomized controlled trial to explore the efficacy and safety of transcranial direct current stimulation on patients with post-stroke fatigue. *Medicine*, 100(41), e27504. https://doi.org/10.1097/MD.0000000000027504

Gaede, G., Tiede, M., Lorenz, I., Brandt, A. U., Pfueller, C., Dörr, J., . . . Paul, F. (2017). Safety and preliminary efficacy of deep transcranial magnetic stimulation in MS-related fatigue. *Neurology, Neuroimmunology & Neuroinflammation*, 5 (1). https://doi.org/10.1212/NXI.00000 00000000423

Glavå, G., & Johansson, B. (2025). Mindfulness-based stress reduction as perceived by individuals with pathological mental fatigue after an acquired brain injury. *Scientific Reports*, 15, 6680. https://doi.org/ 10.1038/s41598-025-90452-y

Glavå, G., Rönnbäck, L., & Johansson, B. (2025). A new mindfulness and psycho-educative program for treatment of brain fatigue, evaluated after an acquired brain injury and multiple sclerosis. *Health Psychology and Behavioral Medicine*, 13(1), 2502039. https://doi.org/10.1080/21642 850.2025.2502039

Grossman, P., Kappos, L., Gensicke, H., D'Souza, M., Mohr, D. C., Penner, I. K., & Steiner, C. (2010). MS quality of life, depression, and fatigue improve after mindfulness training: A randomized trial. *Neurology*, 75(13), 1141–1149.

Grossman, P., Niemannb, L., Schmidtc, S., & Walachc, H. (2004). Mindfulness-based stress reduction and health benefits: A meta-analysis. *Journal of Psychosomatic Research*, 57(2004), 35–43, 57.

Hammett, S. T., Cook, E., Hassan, O., Hughes, C.-A., Rooslien, H., Tizkar, R., & Larsson, J. (2020). GABA, noise and gain in human visual cortex. *Neuroscience Letters*, 736(135294). https://doi.org/10. 1016/j.neulet.2020.135294

Howard, A. (2021). *Decode Your Fatigue*. Hay House Publishers.

Jha, A., Weintraub, A., Allshouse, A., Morey, C., Cusick, C., Kittelson, J., . . . Gerber, D. (2008). A randomized trial of modafinil for the treatment of fatigue and excessive daytime sleepiness in individuals with chronic traumatic brain injury. *Journal of Head Trauma Rehabilitation*, 23(1), 52–63.

Johansson, B., Andréll, P., Rönnbäck, L., & Mannheimer, C. (2020). Follow-up after 5.5 years of treatment with methylphenidate for mental fatigue and cognitive function after a mild traumatic brain injury. *Brain Injury*, 34(2), 229–235. https://doi.org/10.1080/02699052.2019.1683898

Johansson, B., Bjuhr, H., Karlsson, M., Karlsson, J.-O., & Rönnbäck, L. (2015a). Mindfulness-based stress reduction (MBSR) delivered live on the internet to individuals suffering from mental fatigue after an acquired brain injury. *Mindfulness*, 6, 1356–1365.

Johansson, B., Bjuhr, H., & Rönnbäck, L. (2012a). Mindfulness based stress reduction improves long-term mental fatigue after stroke or traumatic brain injury. *Brain Injury*, 26(13–14), 1621–1628.

Johansson, B., Bjuhr, H., & Rönnbäck, L. (2015b). Evaluation of an advanced mindfulness program following a mindfulness-based stress reduction program for participants suffering from mental fatigue after acquired brain injury. *Mindfulness*, 6(2), 227–233. https://doi. org/10.1007/s12671-013-0249-z

Johansson, B., Carlsson, A., Carlsson, M. L., Karlsson, M., Nilsson, M. K. L., Nordquist-Brandt, E., & Rönnbäck, L. (2012b). Placebo-controlled cross-over study of the monoaminergic stabiliser (−)-OSU6162 in mental fatigue following stroke or traumatic brain injury. *Acta Neuropsychiatrica*, 24(5), 266–274.

Johansson, B., & Dalhielm, E. (2024). An online self-study mindfulness-based stress reduction course for people suffering from mental fatigue after an acquired brain injury. *Brain Injury*, 27. https://doi.org/10.1080/02699052.2024.2347545

Johansson, B., Wentzel, A.-P., Andréll, P., Mannheimer, C., & Rönnbäck, L. (2015c). Methylphenidate reduces mental fatigue and improves processing speed in persons suffered a traumatic brain injury. *Brain Injury*, 29(6), 758–765.

Johansson, B., Wentzel, A.-P., Andréll, P., Odenstedt, J., Mannheimer, C., & Rönnbäck, L. (2014). Evaluation of dosage, safety and effects of methylphenidate on posttraumatic brain injury symptoms with focus on mental fatigue and pain. *Brain Injury*, 28(3), 304–310.

Kabat-Zinn, J. (2001). *Full Full catastrophe living: How to Cope with Stress, Pain and Illness Using Mindfulness Meditation*, 15th ed. Piatkus Books.

Kaiser, P. R., Valko, P. O., Werth, E., Thomann, J., Meier, J., Stocker, R., . . . Baumann, C. R. (2010). Modafinil ameliorates excessive daytime sleepiness after traumatic brain injury. *Neurology*, 75(20), 1780–1785.

Kamamuta, A., Takagi, Y., Takahashi, M., Kurihara, K., Shibata, H., Tanaka, K., & Hata, K. (2023). Fatigue potentially reduces the effect of transcranial magnetic stimulation on depression following COVID-19 and its vaccination. *Vaccines*, 25(11), 7. https://doi.org/10.3390/vaccines11071151

Ledineka, A. H., Sajkob, M. C., & Rota, U. (2013). Evaluating the effects of amantadin, modafinil and acetyl-l-carnitine on fatigue in multiple sclerosis – result of a pilot randomized, blind study. *Clinical Neurology and Neurosurgery*, 115(1), S86–S89.

Lezak, M. D., Howieson, D. B., & Loring, D. W. (2004). *Neuropsychological Assessment*, 4th ed. Oxford University Press.

Lutz, A., Jha, A. P., Dunne, J. D., & Saron, C. D. (2015). Investigating the phnomenological matrix of mindfulnessrelated practices from neurocognitive perspective. *American Psychologist*, 70(7), 632–658.

Lutz, A., Slagter, H. A., Dunne, J. D., & Davidson, R. J. (2008). Attention regulation and monitoring in meditation. *Trends in Cognitive Sciences*, 12(4), 163–169.

McKechnie, F. (2023). *Mindfulness-Based Therapy for Managing Fatigue Supporting People with ME/CFS, Fibromyalgia and Long Covid.* Jessica Kingsley Publishers.

Nguyen, S., McKay, A., Wong, D., Rajaratnam, S. M., Spitz, G., Williams, G., . . . Ponsford, J. L. (2017). Cognitive behavior therapy to treat sleep disturbance and fatigue after traumatic brain injury: A pilot randomized controlled trial. *Archives of Physical Medicine and Rehabilitation*, 98(8), 1508–1517.

Nilsson, M. K. L., Johansson, B., Carlsson, M. L., Schuit, R. C., & Rönnbäck, L. (2020). Effect of the monoaminergic stabiliser (−)-OSU6162 on mental fatigue following stroke or traumatic brain injury.

Acta Neuropsychiatrica, 32(6), 303–312. https://doi.org/10.1017/neu.2020.22

Nourbakhsh, B., Revirajan, N., Morris, B., Cordano, C., Creasman, J., Manguinao, M., . . . Waubant, E. (2021). Safety and efficacy of amantadine, modafinil, and methylphenidate for fatigue in multiple sclerosis: A randomised, placebo-controlled, crossover, double-blind trial. *Lancet Neurology*, 20(1), P38–48.

Packer, T. L., Brink, N., & Sauriol, A. (1995). *Managing Fatigue – A Six-Week Course for Energy Conservation*. Therapy Skill Builders.

Ponsford, J., Lee, N. K., Wong, D., McKay, A., Haines, K., Downing, M., . . . O'Donnell, M. L. (2020). Factors associated with response to adapted cognitive behavioral therapy for anxiety and depression following traumatic brain injury. *Journal of Head Trauma Rehabilitation*, 35(2), 117–126. https://doi.org/10.1097/HTR.0000000000000510

Sinclair, K. L., Ponsford, J. L., Taffe, J., Lockley, S. W., & Rajaratnam, S. M. (2014). Randomized controlled trial of light therapy for fatigue following traumatic brain injury. *Neurorehabilitation & Neural Repair*, 28(4), 303–313.

Stankoff, B., Waubant, E., Confavreux, C., Edan, G., Debouverie, M., Rumbach, L., . . . Clanet, M. (2005). Modafinil for fatigue in MS, a randomized placebo-controlled double-blind study. *Neurology*, 64(7). https://doi.org/10.1212/01.WNL.0000158272.27070.6A

Tenovuo, O. (2005). Central acetylcholinesterase inhibitors in the treatment of chronic traumatic brain injury – clinical exeperience in 111 patients. *Progress in Neuro-Psychopharmacology and Biological Psychiatry*, 29, 61–67.

Tenovuo, O., Alin, J., & Helenius, H. (2009). A randomized controlled trial of rivastigmine for chronic sequels of traumatic brain injury—What it showed and taught? *Brain Injury*, 23(6), 548–558.

Western, E., Haug Nordenmark, T., Sorteberg, W., Sorteberg, A., Karic, T., & Sorteberg, A. (2021). (−)-OSU6162 in the treatment of fatigue and other sequelae after aneurysmal subarachnoid hemorrhage: A double-blind, randomized, placebo-controlled study. *Journal of Neurosurgery*, 136(6), 1705–1715. https://doi.org/10.3171/2021.7.JNS211305

Zedlitz, A. M. E. E., Rietveld, T. C. M., Geurts, A. C., & Fasotti, L. (2012). Cognitive and graded activity training can alleviate persistent fatigue after stroke. *Stroke*, 43, 1046–1051.

Zhang, W.-T., & Wang, Y.-F. (2017). Efficacy of methylphenidate for the treatment of mental sequelae after traumatic brain injury. *Medicine*, 95(25), e6960.

8 Work and studies

Regardless of the cause of brain fatigue, work and studies can be demanding and often require adaptation. Children and adolescents with congenital conditions or those who have acquired a brain injury during their development and experience brain fatigue need adjustments in school, as well as later in life when entering the workforce.

The following section addresses the challenges of finding suitable employment or returning to work or studies after a period of illness.

Returning to work after experiencing brain fatigue can be a lengthy process, sometimes taking several years. For some individuals, returning to work or even finding a job may never be possible. This uncertainty can be frustrating, especially since we lack reliable prognostic tools. Some people may return to work, even full-time, only to find themselves feeling overwhelmed and exhausted.

Several studies involving participants with brain fatigue from acquired brain injuries and other illnesses show a reduced ability to return to work, even after many years. It has been suggested that fatigue should be routinely screened for, and patients and employers should be informed about its impact on work and studies, as well as returning to work. We agree with this recommendation.

The importance of endurance for work and studies

From clinical experience, patients usually have a strong desire to return to their ordinary lives, including work or studies. However, they may not always accept or understand their reduced capacity. This is also true for many doctors and healthcare providers. The care for chronic and long-term illnesses and reduced mental energy is seldom acknowledged and understood. There is also an economic burden, and the risk that the sick leave suggested by the doctor is not accepted by the social health insurance.

DOI: 10.4324/9781003732105-8

It is difficult for everyone to understand reduced endurance. As described by Muriel Lezak et al. (2004, page 177)

> Activities that are normally automatic but become effortful after the injury include many that are performed frequently throughout a normal day, such as concentrating, warding off distractions, reading for meaning, doing mental calculations, monitoring ongoing performance, planning the day's activities, attending to conversations at once, or conversing with background noise, etc. It is no wonder that by late afternoon, if not by noon, many of these patients are exhausted.
>
> and Luann Jacobs (https://llanojake.wordpress.com/2011/12/16/mild-brain-injury-implications-for-independence/):
>
> Mild brain injury is a real misnomer, as it conveys the idea that nothing much is a problem when quite the opposite is more often true. It is called 'mild' because the mildly brain injured can walk, talk, eat, and dress independently, often drive a car, shop, cook, go to school, or even work. What the term fails to account for is the inherent limits of how often, for how long (endurance), and how consistently (e.g., every day, once a week) these activities can be performed. The fatigue they feel defies description, going far beyond and far deeper than anything a non-brain-injured person would consider profound exhaustion.

Assessment for work ability

A thorough assessment of work ability is necessary, especially for brain fatigue. This includes assessing the ability to repeat activities day after day without total exhaustion. It is not just about function; it is about endurance, well-being, and sustainable everyday living. Many patients work far beyond their capacity, are not on sick leave, and their doctors may not understand their struggles. They work full-time, and this is what the doctor sees: "You can, so what is the problem?" But many struggle immensely, feeling unsupported and without help from healthcare. Some reduce their working hours without compensation. Those who struggle too hard with work often leave household responsibilities to their partners, if possible, and have little energy left for family, friends, and leisure activities. Parents with children who need care find this very frustrating, as they cannot be the parents they wish to be.

The idea that returning to work will help recovery is not applicable to brain fatigue. The opposite is true. It is not possible to push oneself beyond the personal energy budget. Starting work too early can lead to worsening brain fatigue and total exhaustion later (Figure 8.1, solid black line). A reduction in working hours or complete sick leave may be needed.

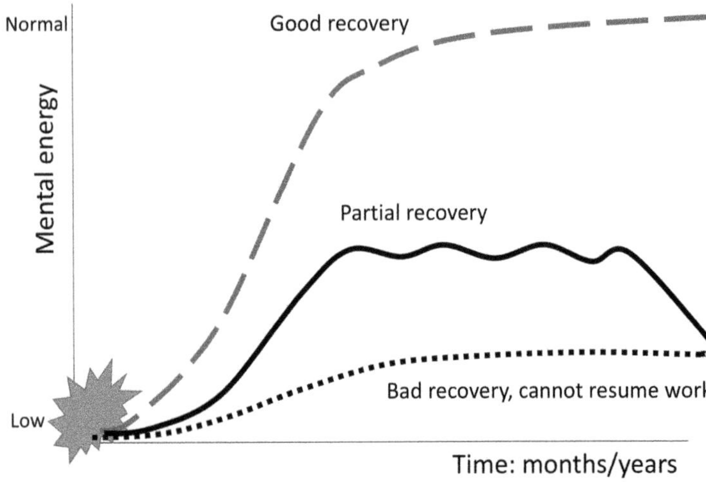

Figure 8.1 The figure shows what can happen after a brain injury, here exemplified by a mild brain injury (grey star at the bottom left in the figure). Most people who have experienced a mild head injury from a medical point of view recover completely and do not have any problems with brain fatigue (grey dashed line). A small proportion (black dotted line) have major problems and do not return to work or normal social life due to brain fatigue after the head injury. A third group (black solid line) regains some mental energy and returns to work and social activities, but not totally. However, after some time, if the activity level is not adapted, they notice that the brain fatigue becomes worse and they need to decrease their working hours. This is important to avoid, and careful follow-up is therefore important for the patient.

However, with knowledge and care, total exhaustion can be avoided. Since there is currently no treatment or method to speed up recovery, returning to work must be done carefully, prioritizing well-being and quality of life.

Time to go back to work

After a period of rehabilitation and recovery, it may be time to consider going back to work or studies. It feels better, the brain fatigue is reduced, and it is possible to be more active at home as well as outside the home. Then, an assessment of work ability needs to be done. If it shows that it is possible to resume work or studies, it is important to do that carefully. Great consideration must be given to mental endurance, as to how the activity can be processed over the entire working day, the next day, next week, and next month. In addition, life outside work must also be included in the evaluation of work ability, as well as the transportation back and forth to work. All consume mental energy.

Work, whatever it is, takes a lot of energy, but to varying degrees. All work requires thinking, concentration, planning and organization and are filled with impressions. In addition, most work must be performed within a certain time frame, with demands on efficiency. It is not about competence level and education. Even jobs that do not require any special education are energy demanding.

Children and adults can also suffer from brain fatigue. However, the younger the child, the harder it is for the child to explain difficulties, but the same consideration and care when going back to school is needed, in the same way as for adults going back to work.

Screening for brain fatigue and work ability

We have evaluated a screening method using the self-report scales Work Ability Index (WAI) and Mental Fatigue Scale (MFS). In the study, we included three diagnostic groups who are commonly affected by brain fatigue: acquired brain injury (traumatic brain injury and stroke), burnout syndrome, and hypothyroidism (thyroid hormone deficiency). All groups commonly report fatigue and are common in primary care. The results showed a significant relationship between WAI and MFS and status in the workplace. Status in the workplace was reported as the working hours in percentage in relation to fulltime employment (in Sweden, 40h/week). We also showed WAI and MFS to be significant predictors for status in the workplace.

This screening method can help healthcare professionals identify individuals with brain fatigue and reduced work ability who need a thorough investigation. For example, if someone has an MFS score above 20 and a poor WAI index, work may not be appropriate yet. Other health-related issues should also be considered in an in-depth work ability assessment. While we cannot provide specific figures for when it is possible to work part-time or full-time, this screening method can guide workplace adaptations.

The screening method can also be used for follow-up when work has resumed or when working hours are increased. It is important to ensure that brain fatigue does not increase, as indicated by the dotted line in Figure 8.2. Ideally, brain fatigue should remain stable or decrease, following the solid arrow.

Using the MFS and WAI questionnaires can help individuals become aware of their actual situation. These questionnaires encourage self-reflection about work, life, and mental energy, which is important.

This screening method enables early rehabilitation and preventive action for individuals affected by illnesses that cause brain fatigue. It helps prevent exhaustion, either before resuming work or for those already working but experiencing signs of fatigue. The goal is always to promote a sustainable and well-functioning workplace and the well-being of the individual.

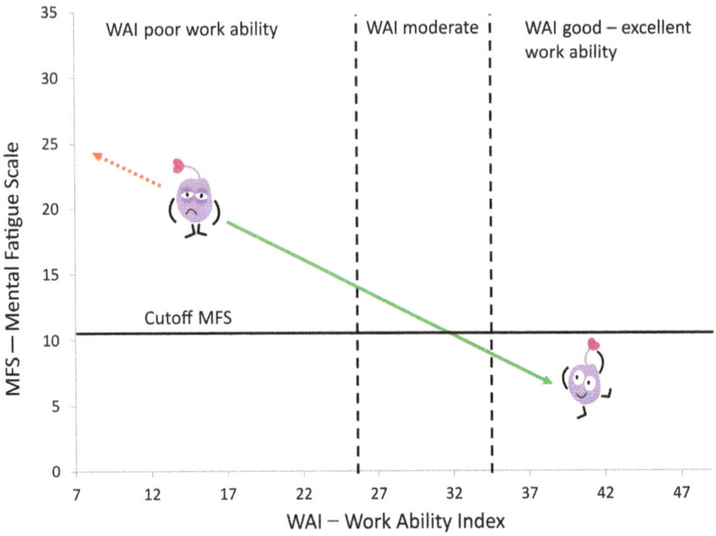

Figure 8.2 Screening work ability with MFS and WAI. The Mental Fatigue Scale (MFS) and Work Ability Index (WAI) can be used as screening tools for assessing work ability and for follow-up evaluations. This diagram illustrates how a person reports brain fatigue and work ability. These initial screenings should be followed by an in-depth work ability assessment. For future planning, it is crucial to avoid the dotted line, which indicates increased brain fatigue, and aim to follow the solid arrow, which shows reduced brain fatigue. The WAI is divided into poor, moderate, and good-to-excellent categories, indicated by longitudinal dashed lines, while the MFS indicates brain fatigue above the cutoff (horizontal line).

How to resume work

Returning to work or starting a new job needs to be planned collaboratively with all involved. Discussions should focus on what can be done to make it possible. Sometimes, returning to the old job may not be feasible if it cannot be adapted or if there is no job to return to. Seeking help from professionals, employers, organizations, and healthcare providers is recommended. Generally, people with brain fatigue are ambitious and want to be more active than their energy budget allows. It is important to remember that individuals returning to work after a long sick leave still, to some extent, suffer from brain fatigue. Part-time work is recommended initially.

When resuming work, it should be done in small steps with time for rest. Initially, having a full day off between workdays can help with energy recovery. Work should be adapted to be calmer, in a quiet place, doing one task at a time, and using other useful strategies based on personal resources

Table 8.1 Example of a weekly schedule with days for rest and recovery. For some, a few hours of work every day is best. It all depends on the job and how tiring the commute is

% Of full-time work (%)	*Monday*	*Tuesday*	*Wednesday*	*Thursday*	*Friday*
25	4 h	Rest	3 h	Rest	3 h
25	2 h	2 h	2 h	2 h	2 h
50	5 h	5 h	Rest	5 h	5 h
75	7.5 h	7.5 h	Rest	7.5 h	7.5 h
75	6 h	6 h	6 h	6 h	6 h

and the workplace. A quiet and calm place for rest is desirable. Starting with familiar tasks based on routines and previous experiences is often best, as learning new tasks and routines requires a lot of energy. For some, trying a different job may be a good idea if returning to the old job is not suitable. Working every day may be possible for some but not for others. Working from home can be beneficial from time to time if possible. There is no one-size-fits-all template. Work should also be adapted to the energy demands of the commute. Resting before starting the workday may be necessary if the commute is long. Quiet lunch breaks are helpful for most. An individual schedule that provides the best possible return to work is beneficial, as exemplified in Table 8.1.

Resuming studies is just as demanding. Studying part-time can be difficult but desirable. Studies must be adapted to the individual's needs, such as taking fewer courses, extending the duration of studies, or considering distance learning.

Bibliography

Andersen, G., Christensen, D., Kirkevold, M., & Johnsen, S. P. (2012). Post-stroke fatigue and return to work: A 2-year follow-up. *Acta Neurologica Scandinavica*, 125(4), 248–253. https://doi.org/10.1111/j.1600-0404.2011.01557.x Epub 2011 Jun 21.

Fahrenfort, J. J., Wilterdink, A. M. L., & van der Veen, E. A. (2000). Long-term residual complaints and psychosocial sequelae after remission of hyperthyroidism. *Psychoneuroendocrinology*, 25, 201–211.

Johansson, B. (2022). Screening method for assessment of work ability for patients suffering from mental fatigue. *Frontiers in Behavioral Neuroscience*, 16, 869377. https://doi.org/10.3389/fnbeh.2022.869377

Lezak, M. D., Howieson, D. B., & Loring, D. W. (2004). *Neuropsychological Assessment*, 4th ed., Oxford University Press.

Norlander, A., Lindgren, I., Pessah-Rasmussen, H., Gard, G., & Brogårdh, C. (2021). Fatigue in men and women who have returned to work after stroke: Assessed with the fatigue severity scale and mental

fatigue scale. *Journal of Rehabilitation Medicine*, 9(53), jrm00227. https://doi.org/10.2340/16501977-2863
Palm, S., Rönnbäck, L., & Johansson, B. (2017). Long-term mental fatigue after traumatic brain injury and impact on capacity for workemployment status. *Journal of Rehabilitation Mededicine*, 49, 228–233.
Waljas, M., Iverson, G. L., Lange, R. T., Liimatainen, S., Hartikainen, K. M., Dastidar, P., . . . Öhman, J. (2014). Return to work following mild traumatic brain injury. *Journal of Head Trauma Rehabilitation*, 29(5), 443–450.

9 And then

To mourn what has been lost

When people suffer from injuries and illnesses that cause long-term brain fatigue, it often leads to frustration and sadness over activities and relationships that no longer function as they once did. Memory fails, attention is hard to maintain, and returning to work or continuing studies becomes difficult or impossible. Spending time with family and friends, despite the strong desire to do so, becomes very strenuous. This often results in cancelled meetings with loved ones, not due to a lack of will, but due to a lack of energy and the ability to manage the overwhelming impressions. Knowing that such meetings will lead to exhaustion and require a long recovery period sets limits on life. This can make life lonely and many feel isolated from everyday activities.

Brain fatigue is a hidden condition. People around those suffering from it often struggle to understand how it feels. This lack of understanding is often reinforced by preconceived notions about how things should be. We judge and evaluate without truly knowing the experience. We need to listen and learn from those suffering from brain fatigue, approaching with curiosity and an open mind, without ready-made solutions, but with a genuine interest in understanding deeper.

People suffering from brain fatigue often have a strong desire to be "normal" and participate in life. Many try repeatedly, with excursions, travels, or dinners, but fall back into exhaustion and disappointment. This leads to growing frustration and grief, and there is an increased risk of depression. Anxiety can also develop when it becomes difficult to handle a large amount of unsorted impressions and being easily disturbed.

Included in society

When life changes drastically, it affects not only the person but also everyone around them. No one lives in complete isolation. Everyone wants to be included and integrated into society, woven together with others.

DOI: 10.4324/9781003732105-9

It can be challenging for a person with brain fatigue to share life with their partner, parents, and children, and maintain contact with friends. They want to, but can't manage. For relatives and friends, the change in life can also be difficult to manage when everyday activities can no longer be shared as before. Relatives may grieve over shared activities that no longer work, especially when brain fatigue becomes long-lasting or chronic.

If there are children in the family, adjustments must be made. Children have their needs and require parental attention. Being a parent with brain fatigue and facing this reality is difficult. The child still needs support and help, which cannot be neglected, placing an extra burden on the other parent or others who can provide support.

Partners, family members, or close friends can sometimes be the ones who most clearly see the difficulties arising for the person with brain fatigue and can suggest rest when needed. When the situation is reversed, and partners, family, and friends do not fully understand, it may lead to excessive demands on the person with brain fatigue, resulting in irritation and conflicts.

Since most people do not live in complete isolation but in a relational context, everyone is affected, and all close ones also need support in the new life situation.

To meet life on its own terms

When something drastic happens, the wish is often to regain the old life. However, this may not be possible. Understanding how life is now, no matter how tough and difficult, is important for building the "new life."

Several years ago, we started a Facebook group for brain fatigue. The purpose was to share experiences, provide support, and not feel alone. This is expressed here:

> I am practicing letting go of resistance. Resistance to the change that has remained. I have mourned for a long time the person I once was, for she will never return. But something has happened to me when I stopped resisting. I meet a new person, and she is me. Vulnerable, forgetful, and sometimes incredibly tired. I was long cemented in resistance. Slowly, I am breaking free. It is difficult, and there are no manuals. So I practice and am immensely grateful to practice together with you. Because we are creating the manual together.

Acceptance does not mean giving up but becoming fully aware of the difficulties and possibilities that exist. It means understanding the reality and

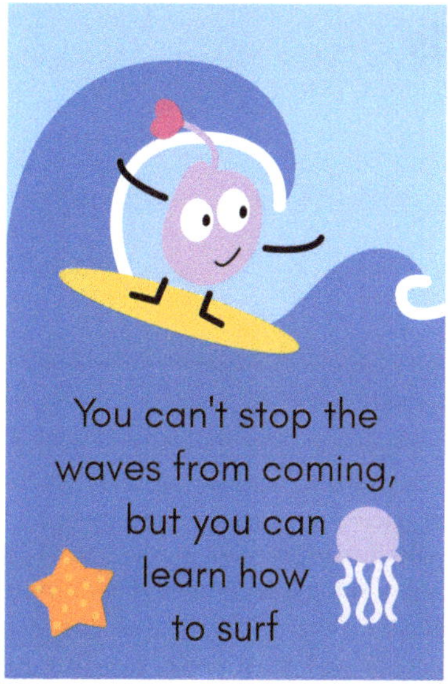
You can't stop the
waves from coming,
but you can
learn how
to surf

Figure 9.1 Acceptance.

meeting life with courage. This awareness provides the opportunity to choose and perhaps take a new path.

Difficulties are a part of life, but how we manage them determines whether they take over our lives or whether we can handle them more easily. It may feel impossible, but working on how we meet and cope with life is possible. This can involve discovering new ways to relate to oneself, thinking about oneself, or reacting and dealing with difficult situations (Figure 9.1).

> I think part of accepting is just accepting that life did not turn out as I had imagined. I mourned for a long time what I lost until one day I began to look ahead. What has happened cannot be changed. Then to find hope and joy again is actually possible. I became who I became and am who I am. Some days are crap, just like life was before. But I'm different and I like the one I became.

Final words

Brain fatigue syndrome needs to be understood by everyone. It is not sustainable to push through work, studies, and leisure activities at an increasingly hectic and fast pace. For those affected by brain fatigue, it becomes difficult to participate in society with studies, work, and social life in a desirable way, and there is a risk that mental health will deteriorate.

We need to understand the significance of energy deficiency in determining what is possible and reasonable, not just what is desirable or expected by society. The unknown, invisible, and difficult-to-understand must be brought to the surface and made comprehensible.

We propose a collective term for this lack of energy: Brain Fatigue Syndrome, BFS. This symptom complex, with energy depletion as the overarching feature, is common to many different diseases and conditions that affect the brain.

When a person exhibits symptoms of BFS, it indicates that the brain is affected by disease or injury. While many consider these symptoms to be non-specific, we believe they provide evidence of brain impact due to injury, disease, or systemic inflammation, including autoimmunity. These conditions, whether they directly affect the brain or result from bodily disease impacting the brain via the blood-brain barrier, lead to inflammatory activation of astrocytes. These inflammatory-reactive astrocytes give rise to disturbed neuronal signalling, even if the neurones themselves may not necessarily be damaged or disturbed in function. Therefore, BFS does not always signify specific nerve cell damage but rather a secondary effect of a nerve cell disorder. In our view, symptoms within BFS are specific indicators of brain impact.

Typical BFS includes reduced endurance and an unusually prolonged recovery of mental energy, even after moderate cognitive exertion. Affected individuals often experience a persistent lack of energy, which becomes particularly noticeable during mental activities. This energy deficit is likely apparent to both the affected person and those around them.

DOI: 10.4324/9781003732105-10

Emotional symptoms, such as increased emotionality and irritability, are also common. Another significant issue is the inability to filter out irrelevant information, such as sounds and lights. For example, the noise from a low-frequency fan or car traffic outside can continuously disturb the person affected by brain fatigue. Normally, our brains filter out these sounds, reducing strain. The real problem is that their brains are overloaded and easily distracted by redundant information, limiting their ability to focus on tasks. This distraction may lead to information loss during conversations.

The lack of mental energy contributes to the inability of those affected to work in open labour markets. People sometimes suggest "simpler" jobs, assuming they require less cognitive capacity. However, this assumption is flawed. Many individuals with brain fatigue have good cognitive functions in terms of information intake, processing, and memory storage.

To summarize, BFS may be a manifestation of brain damage, a neurological disease, or a systemic illness that affects the brain, such as a severe infection or inflammation. It can also occur as a side effect of certain medical treatments.

Today, BFS can be alleviated; methods do exist, although none are miraculous. This is not insignificant, as many individuals actively seek help. Employing approaches that support people in adapting to their actual energy levels and understanding the impact of BFS on their well-being can assist them in their efforts to find new ways of living. Support may be needed from time to time, as the process is often long and marked by fluctuations.

We must approach people with Brain Fatigue Syndrome with an open mind and curiosity, avoiding preconceived notions about tiredness. Only then can we provide adequate support for those suffering from Brain Fatigue Syndrome.

Appendix

Mental Fatigue Scale, MFS

Name:________________________ Date: ______________

We are interested in *your present condition*, that is, how you have felt during *the past month*.

When you are comparing your condition with "than before", compare it with how it was before the injury or getting ill.

Each question below is followed by four statements that describe: No (0), Slight (1), Fairly serious (2) and Serious (3) problems. We would like you to place a circle around the figure before the statement that best describes your problems. Should you find that your problem falls between two statements, there are also figures to indicate this.

---

1. **Fatigue**
   Have you felt fatigued during the past month? It does not matter if the fatigue is physical (muscular) or mental. If you recently experienced something unusual (for example an accident or short illness) you should try to disregard it when assessing your fatigue.

0	I do not feel fatigued at all. (No abnormal fatigue, do not need to rest more than usual).
0.5	
1	I feel fatigued several times every day but I feel more alert after a rest.
1.5	
2	I feel fatigued for most of the day and taking a rest has little or no effect.
2.5	
3	I feel fatigued all the time and taking a rest makes no difference.

2. **Lack of initiative**
   Do you find it difficult to start things? Do you experience resistance or a lack of initiative when you have to start something, no matter whether it is a new task or part of your everyday activities?

0	I have no difficulty starting things.
0.5	
1	I find it more difficult starting things than I used to. I'd rather do it some other time.
1.5	
2	It takes a great effort to start things. This applies to everyday activities such as getting out of bed, washing myself and eating.
2.5	
3	I can't do the simplest of everyday tasks (eating, getting dressed). I need help with everything.

3. **Mental fatigue**
   Does your brain become fatigued quickly when you have to think hard? Do you become mentally fatigued from things such as reading, watching TV or taking part in a conversation with several people? Do you have to take breaks or change to another activity?

0	I can manage in the same way as usual. My ability for sustained mental effort is not reduced.
0.5	
1	I become fatigued quickly but am still able to make the same mental effort as before.
1.5	
2	I become fatigued quickly and have to take a break or do something else more often than before.
2.5	
3	I become fatigued so quickly that I can do nothing or have to abandon everything after a short period (approx. five minutes).

4. **Mental recovery**
   How long do you need to recover after you have worked "until you drop" or are no longer able to concentrate on what you are doing?

0	I need to rest for less than an hour before continuing whatever I am doing.
0.5	
1	I need to rest for more than an hour but do not require a night's sleep.
1.5	
2	I need a night's sleep before I can continue whatever I am doing.
2.5	
3	I need several days rest in order to recover.

5. **Concentration difficulties**
   Do you find it difficult to gather your thoughts and concentrate?

0	I can concentrate as usual.
0.5	
1	I sometimes lose concentration, for example when reading or watching TV.
1.5	
2	I find it so difficult to concentrate that I have problems, for example reading a newspaper or taking part in a conversation with a group of people.
2.5	
3	I always have such difficulty concentrating that it is almost impossible to do anything.

6. **Memory problems**
   Do you forget things more often than before, do you need to make notes or do you have to search for things at home or at work?

0	I have no memory problems.
0.5	
1	I forget things slightly more often than I should, but I am able to manage by making notes.
1.5	
2	My poor memory causes frequent problems (for example forgetting important meetings or turning off the cooker).
2.5	
3	I can hardly remember anything at all.

7. **Slowness of thinking**
   Do you feel slow or sluggish when you think about something? Do you feel that it takes an unusually long time to conclude a train of thought or solve a task that requires mental effort?

0	My thoughts are neither slow nor sluggish when it comes to work involving mental effort.
0.5	
1	My thoughts are a bit slow one or a few times each day when I have to do something that requires serious mental effort.
1.5	
2	My thoughts often feel slow and sluggish, even when carrying out everyday activities, for example a conversation with a person or when reading the newspaper.
2.5	
3	My thoughts always feel very slow and sluggish.

8. **Sensitivity to stress**
Do you find it difficult to cope with stress that is, doing several things at the same time while under time pressure?

0	I am able to cope with stress, in the same way as usual.
0.5	
1	I become more easily stressed, but only in demanding situations that I was previously able to manage.
1.5	
2	I become stressed more easily than before. I feel stressed in situations that previously did not bother me.
2.5	
3	I become stressed very easily. I feel stressed in unfamiliar or trying situations.

9. **Increased tendency to become emotional**
Do you find that you cry more easily than previously? Do you often burst into tears when, for example, you watch a sad film or talk with your family members? If you recently experienced something unusual (e.g. an accident or short illness) you should try to disregard it in your assessment.

0	I am not more emotional than I used to be.
0.5	
1	I am more emotional than other people but it is something that is natural for me. I start to cry or my eyes fill with tears easily, but only in relation to things that affect me deeply.
1.5	
2	My emotions are problematic or embarrassing. I sometimes even start to cry about things that mean nothing to me. I try to avoid certain situations because of this.
2.5	
3	My emotions cause me great problems. They disturb my day-to-day relationship with members of my immediate family and make it difficult for me to cope outside the home.

10. **Irritability or "a short fuse"**
Are you unusually short-tempered or irritable about things that previously did not bother you?

0	I am not more short-tempered or irritable than I used to be.
0.5	
1	I become more easily irritated, but it does not last very long.
1.5	
2	I become irritated very quickly about small things or things that do not bother other people.
2.5	
3	I react with extreme anger or rage, which I find very difficult to control.

11. **Sensitivity to light**
Are you sensitive to strong light?

0	I have no increased sensitivity to light.
0.5	
1	I sometimes experience problems with strong light such as sunlight reflected by snow, water or glass, or strong lights at home, but I am able to cope with it, for example by wearing sunglasses.
1.5	
2	I am so sensitive to light that I prefer to carry out my daily activities in dim light. I find it difficult to leave the house without sunglasses.
2.5	
3	My sensitivity to light is so strong that I am unable to leave the house without sunglasses. I keep the blinds (or equivalent) drawn at all times.

12. **Sensitivity to noise**
Are you sensitive to noise?

0	I do not suffer from increased sensitivity to noise.
0.5	
1	I sometimes have difficulty with loud noise (for example music, noise from the TV or radio or sudden, unexpected sounds), but I can deal with it easily by turning down the volume. My sensitivity to noise does not disturb my everyday life.
1.5	
2	I have a marked over-sensitivity to noise. I have to avoid loud noise or reduce it (for example by means of ear plugs) in order to cope with everyday life.
2.5	
3	My sensitivity to noise is so great that I find it difficult to manage at home despite sound insulation.

13. **Decreased sleep at night**
Do you sleep badly at night? If you are sleeping more than before at night, please place a circle around the "0". If you are taking sleeping tablets and sleep normally, please place a circle around "0".

0	I do not sleep less than before.
0.5	
1	I have slight problems falling asleep or my sleep is shorter, lighter or more restless than before.
1.5	
2	I sleep at least two hours less than before and wake up frequently during the night without anything disturbing me.
2.5	
3	I sleep less than two to three hours per night.

14. **Increased sleep**
Do you sleep longer and/or more deeply than before? If you are sleeping less than before, please place a circle around the "0". N.B. Please take account of time spent sleeping during the day.

0	I do not sleep more than usual.
0.5	
1	I sleep longer or deeper, but less than two hours more than usual, including naps during the day.
1.5	
2	I sleep longer or deeper. At least two hours more than usual, including naps.
2.5	
3	I sleep longer or deeper. At least four hours more than usual, and in addition I need to take a nap during the day.

Total score of item 1–14. A cutoff score at 10.5 is suggested. A score above 10 implicates problems with mental fatigue and the person should consider the actual situation with work or social life.

24-hour variations (for clinical use). Do you find that at certain times of the day or night the problems we asked about (for example tiredness, lack of concentration) are better or worse? In the statements below, "regularly" means at least 3–4 days of the week.

0	I have not noticed that my problems are regularly better or worse at certain times, or I do not have any specific problems.
1	There is a clear difference between certain times of the day. I can predict that I will feel better at certain times and worse at other times.
2	I feel unwell at all times of the day and night.

If you experience 24-hour variations:

When do you feel at your best?	Morning	Afternoon	Evening	Night
When do you feel at your worst?	Morning	Afternoon	Evening	Night

More information about MFS is available at www.brainfatigue.se

Index

Pages in *italics* refer to figures and pages in **bold** refer to tables.

www.ingramcontent.com/pod-product-compliance
Ingram Content Group UK Ltd.
Pitfield, Milton Keynes, MK11 3LW, UK
UKHW022344190926
475702UK00015B/2089
9781041224006